THE DESIGN AND CONSTRUCTION OF REMOVABLE ORTHODONTIC APPLIANCES

By

C. PHILIP ADAMS

M.D.S., F.D.S., D.Orth., R.C.S. Eng., F.F.D. R.C.S.I.

Reader in Orthodontics, Queen's University, Belfast; Consultant in Orthodontics, Belfast Teaching Hospitals. Formerly Lecturer in Orthodontics, School of Dental Surgery, Liverpool; Lecturer in the Department of Orthodontics, Institute of Dental Surgery, British Postgraduate Medical Federation, University of London

490 *Photographs and Diagrams*

FOURTH EDITION

BALTIMORE

THE WILLIAMS AND WILKINS COMPANY

1970

Distribution by Sole Agents:
United States of America: The Williams & Wilkins Company, Baltimore
Canada: The Macmillan Company of Canada, Ltd., Toronto

First edition	1955
Reprinted	1956
Second edition	1957
Reprinted	1959
Reprinted	1961
Third edition	1964
Fourth edition	1970

Italian, Spanish, and French translations have also been made.

ISBN 0 7236 0262 X

PRINTED IN GREAT BRITAIN BY JOHN WRIGHT & SONS LTD., AT THE STONEBRIDGE PRESS, BRISTOL BS4 5NU

PREFACE TO THE FOURTH EDITION

THE preparation of this new edition has entailed a considerable revision of the existing text with clarification and expansion of the subject matter where it has appeared necessary and the addition of a large number of new illustrations. The effects of these rearrangements will be seen especially in connexion with clasp design and construction, the construction of extra-oral traction devices, and orthodontic wire bending technique. A number of additional appliances have been described and illustrated.

The appendices, which in previous editions contained information concerning orthodontic materials, have been brought together and expanded to make a new chapter. The chapter on orthodontic technique has been enlarged with new illustrations which render more explicit points which were previously discussed as matters of general principle.

The chapter on Functional Appliances has been considerably enlarged by the inclusion of a section on the Function Corrector. I wish to express my thanks to Dr. Rolf Fränkel for permission to quote freely from his writings in the *Transactions of the European Orthodontic Society*, 1966. I also wish to thank the European Orthodontic Society for permission to use this material and also to include my own paper "An Investigation into Indications for and the Effects of the Function Regulator" read to the Society at its Conference in Edinburgh, in 1969.

With some reluctance, a slight change in terminology has now been adopted in that "Adams clasp", "Adams universal pliers", and "Adams spring-forming pliers" are used in reference to what were formerly "modified arrowhead clasp", "universal pliers", and "spring-forming pliers". It is not that I have sought to become an eponym but rather that the alteration is in agreement with terminology that has become hallowed by tradition over a period of two decades. Furthermore, the clasp and pliers in question have been carefully specified, described, and illustrated and in the light of experience it has been found that changes and modifications in the designs are not required. It is my hope that when the terms "Adams clasp" and "Adams pliers" are used they will imply agreement with the descriptions that have been given of these appliances and instruments.

I am again indebted to many people who have helped in the preparation of this new edition and I wish especially to thank the following: Dr. W. Russell Logan gave much of his time to introduce me to the uses of the Function Corrector and I spent a most interesting and instructive week at his clinic. Mr. Hill Mercer constructed all the appliances for the new illustrations. Mrs. Carmel Dowd and Miss Vivien Sloan assisted in the preparation of the text and Mrs. Pamela Pollock in the preparation of the new photographs. I also wish to thank many colleagues and members of staff who helped by the treatment of patients and by demonstrating procedures for the illustrations; my wife for support and encouragement throughout the work of this edition; and Mr. L. G. Owens, B.Sc., of John Wright & Sons Ltd., for his patience and help in the production of the volume.

March, 1970   C. P. A.

PREFACE TO THE FIRST EDITION

It is the object of this book to try to establish a systematic approach to the construction of removable orthodontic appliances and at the same time to discuss their usefulness and limitations so that they may be placed in their proper relationship to the other means and techniques that are available for the mechanical treatment of irregularity and malocclusion of the teeth.

The book is based on a series of articles, published originally in the *Dental Practitioner*, which dealt with the mechanical principles of orthodontic appliances in general and the design of removable appliances in particular; the soldering of stainless steel for removable appliance construction and the preparation of coil springs. To this material has now been added a fresh chapter discussing the several factors which affect the design and construction of a removable appliance, with frequent reference to specific examples illustrated in other parts of the book; and chapters on the problems of orthodontic technique and on the design and construction of orthodontic clasps, which embody the essential points and illustrations of articles previously published in the *Dental Record*.

In order to emphasize that appliances are only a means to an end, the sections on appliance construction have been dealt with under the headings of types of tooth movement rather than under any attempted classification of appliance types. Many of the well-known "types" of appliance are no more than mentioned in principle, in the belief that if the principles of their action are understood, the application of these principles can be worked out and applied in practice if required.

It is my belief that the adoption of this approach, based on the consideration of underlying principles, is more flexible and potentially valuable than any listing or description of appliance types. Through this approach it is possible to assess the needs of any given treatment scheme and produce appliances specifically designed to carry out that scheme in the most efficient way.

I am greatly indebted to many people for assistance in the writing of this book and I wish especially to thank:—

Mr. Clifford F. Ballard for his encouragement to embark on this work in the first instance and for his advice and assistance in its furtherance while I was a member of his staff in the Department of Orthodontics, the Institute of Dental Surgery, London.

Mr. H. T. A. McKeag for much helpful advice on the general approach to the subject, and in particular for his comments on the content of Chapters I and II.

Mr. S. G. McCallin for his interest in removable appliances in general, and especially in the development of removable intermaxillary and extra-oral appliances and for permission to reproduce *Figs.* 148, 152, 156, and 157.

Mr. G. G. T. Fletcher for reading Chapter I in manuscript and for his most helpful comments.

Professor H. H. Stones, Mr. J. W. Softley, and the staff of the Orthodontic Department, School of Dental Surgery, Liverpool, for their encouragement and interest in the development of the technique training scheme illustrated in Chapter IV.

Mr. F. D. Rowe, for his suggestion of the Single Arrowhead Clasp (*Fig.* 78), and for preparing the photographs for *Figs.* 39–44 inclusive.

Miss C. C. Jefferson, for suggesting the loop-hook for intermaxillary traction (*Fig.* 76).

Mr. C. V. Hill for the introduction to this country of the cervical traction appliance, *Figs.* 149–152 inclusive.

Mr. J. R. Halden, who developed the technique of soldering fine wires to thick (*Fig.* 237), and who demonstrated this technique to me at the Eastman Dental Hospital, London.

Mr. J. S. Beresford, for a personal communication on the control of boxed-in springs (*Fig.* 16).

Mr. H. L. Parry, B.Sc., for a personal communication on the question of the mechanical action of forces acting on inclined planes.

Mr. D. R. McDougall, F.I.B.P., and his staff of the Department of Photography, Institute of Dental Surgery, London, for the endless care and attention they have given to the preparation of the photographs, and the perfection of the results they have achieved. The photographs for Chapter XVI were taken by myself as, at the time they were required, the services of Mr. McDougall unfortunately were not available to me.

My wife, who has typed the manuscript for publication and who has been a never-failing source of support and encouragement.

Mr. L. G. Owens, B.Sc., of John Wright & Sons Ltd., for his courtesy and help throughout the production of this volume.

The Modified Arrowhead Clasp; the System of Technique Training described in Chapter IV; and Variations of the Modified Arrowhead Clasp were given as demonstrations to the British Society for the Study of Orthodontics at the Demonstration Meetings of the Society in May, 1949, May, 1950, and May, 1954, respectively.

The photographs of appliances in this book are primarily for showing these appliances and the tooth movements they are designed to carry out. It should not be assumed that the cases exemplified by the models used for the illustrations would necessarily be treated in the way that is suggested by the tooth movements being shown. In a few illustrations, appliances are in fact shown on the models of cases which were treated with those appliances.

August, 1955   C. P. A.

CONTENTS

CONTENTS

viii

CHAPTER I

THE MECHANICAL PRINCIPLES OF ORTHODONTIC APPLIANCES

THE reader of orthodontic literature, particularly in England, cannot fail to note the regularity with which "new" appliances and methods for moving teeth are brought forward for his attention and criticism. It is probably true, however, that there is now very little that is basically new in orthodontic technique and that practice swings from one method to another and back again, depending to some extent on contemporary thought and on the personal inclination of the operator in any particular case.

There is no agreement on what appliance is best for use in any given situation, and there is in particular a tendency to think that the user of removable appliances is the "country cousin" of the operator who uses fixed appliances. There can be no doubt, however, that it is better to deal with some situations by fixed appliances and with others by removable appliances for a variety of reasons, and there should be no difficulty in selecting and using the appropriate appliance if the basic principles of design and construction are understood and applied.

THE ACTION OF ORTHODONTIC APPLIANCES

Opinions still differ on how far the influence of appliances extends through the teeth beyond the immediate alveolar bone and produces effects in the more remote parts of the jaws. There can be little doubt that the first and most obvious effect of appliances is to bring pressure or tension to bear on the teeth. This force is in turn transmitted to the bone surrounding the roots of the teeth, producing, on one side of the root, a pressure on the surrounding bone, and, on the other, a tension through the attachment of the tooth to the bone by the periodontal membrane. This pressure and tension on the alveolar bone lead to the processes of bone resorption and deposition which permit tooth movement and remodelling of the bony socket around the root of the tooth as movement takes place.

The action of appliances is most clearly apparent in those appliances which consist of a metal spring under tension, and a framework on which the spring is supported and through which the reaction of the spring is dispersed over the anchorage. Most removable appliances and labiolingual appliances fall into this category.

It is more difficult to analyse the action of such appliances as the twin wire arch, the edgewise arch, and the round wire arch appliances, and to measure the amount and assess the nature of the forces they exert on individual teeth. These appliances are usually attached to all, or nearly all, the teeth in the dental arch, so that complicated anchorage problems may arise in their use. These appliances also have the special property of being able to produce a tipping of the apices of the teeth; the pressure which results from this movement is not easy to assess.

Functional appliances produce pressures on teeth which are difficult to assess because the pressures are derived either directly from the actions of the facial or masticatory muscles or by preventing the action of these muscles from producing pressures upon the teeth. Active pressures produced by such appliances as the Andresen appliance, the bite plane, or the inclined plane can be very large, depending on the exertions of the patient, while such appliances as the oral screen and the function corrector may prevent the tongue, lips, and cheeks from exerting pressures upon the tooth

1

crowns and thereby allow opposing muscular or other influences to produce movements of teeth.

The precise effects of traction and of screw appliances need also to be carefully considered.

THE ACTION OF REMOVABLE AND LABIOLINGUAL APPLIANCES

The action of these appliances is the action of the springs that are used on them. The terms "spring" and "auxiliary spring" are sometimes used synonymously without any real distinction in meaning being made. Strictly speaking, an "auxiliary spring" should be a spring which is separate in construction and used as an aid to some other, larger, pre-existing spring. An "auxiliary spring" is sometimes thought of as a spring attached to an archwire as distinct from a spring attached to a baseplate. Unless the archwire is being used as a source of spring pressure, any spring attached to it must be a "spring" and not an "auxiliary spring". A spring attached to a heavy archwire on a removable appliance must be simply a spring as such arches are usually rigid and are regarded as extensions of the baseplate or framework of the appliance.

In labiolingual technique, even heavy archwires can be used to exert expanding or contracting activity as the arches are reasonably long and correspondingly flexible and may act on a number of teeth. In these circumstances any spring attached to such a heavy archwire can properly be called an "auxiliary spring" designed to produce some tooth movement secondary or incidental to the main movements produced by the archwire itself, and it is probably from these circumstances that the term "auxiliary" spring has gained currency in describing springs attached to removable appliances.

In planning the design and lay-out of springs on an appliance, it is important to design a spring that will exert a suitable pressure★ over

an adequate distance. There is no difficulty in making a spring with a *short* range of action; the problem more often is, within the space limitations imposed by the dental arch and the buccal sulcus, to design a spring with a sufficiently *long* range of action. The spring should also be mechanically simple so that its action is as clear as possible.

The spring that best fulfils these requirements is the finger or cantilever spring fixed at one end and free to move at the other (*Fig. 1 A*). The path of movement of the free end is, for practical purposes, at right angles to the length of the spring itself.

When designing a spring it is necessary to make it of wire of such a length and thickness that the optimum degrees of strength and flexibility are secured for the particular situation that the spring is to work in.† It is important to realize that no wire is too thick or too thin to be used for spring construction, if the following effects of range of action and pressure are borne in mind. A light pressure over however long a range of action is safe and tolerable because the periodontal tissues can sustain the pressure and react in their own time to accommodate the movement of the teeth. A heavy pressure over a long range of action is dangerous because the periodontal tissues cannot react quickly enough to accommodate tooth movement and damage is produced owing to occlusion of the blood-vessels and crushing of the tissues. If, therefore, it is necessary for any reason to use a heavy gauge of wire for a spring it must be arranged that the range of action of the spring and the pressure it exerts are within safe limits.

★ It was found by Schwarz (1931) that the most favourable pressure with which to move a tooth is 20 g. per square centimetre of root area. Translated into terms of teeth this is, for practical purposes, equivalent to not

more than 20 g. per single rooted tooth. In practice it has been found that this pressure may be increased for larger teeth—that is, molars and canines. High pressures will produce tooth movement but not necessarily any more quickly than low pressures. With heavy pressures movement takes place by undermining resorption and is accompanied by resorption of cementum and dentine in many cases.

† The formula $D \propto \dfrac{Pl^3}{t^4}$ expresses the relationship between the amount of deflection D, the pressure P, the length l, and the thickness t, for a cantilever spring of round section. The formula only holds true within the elastic limit of the material of which the spring is made.

Two modifications of the cantilever spring that extend its usefulness are the introduction of a coil at the point of attachment of the spring and the addition of an extra limb, so forming the double cantilever spring.

The introduction of a coil at the point of attachment of the spring has the practical effect of increasing the flexibility or range of action of the spring without increasing its dimensions (*Fig.* 1 B).

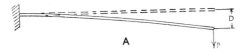

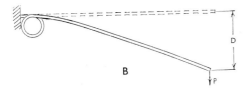

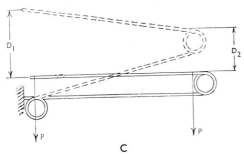

Fig. 1.—The pressure, P, is required to compress these springs to the positions shown by the unbroken lines. The springs then emit this pressure in gradually diminishing amount over the distance, D, D_1 and D_2, as they return to their positions of rest.

In certain circumstances the number of coils may be increased to more than one (*Figs.* 2, 97). In these instances it is important to see that the spring, while increasing its flexibility in the direction of action of the coils, does not become unstable in other directions and hence impractical in use. This drawback may be overcome by providing guides and guards for such springs. It should be remembered also that the addition of too many coils may make the spring so flexible that an excessive amount of deflection may be required before an adequate pressure is built up.

The addition of a second limb to the spring, producing a double cantilever spring, is a modification that is necessary when two or more teeth are to be moved the same distance in

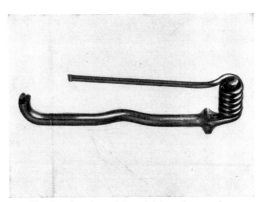

Fig. 2.—A spring with multiple coils wound on a support. This is useful where limitations of space prevent the construction of a longer spring. The spring above is of 0·6-mm. wire, the support of 1·0-mm. wire. The end of the spring is looped around the support and soldered before the coils are wound. (*See Figs.* 96, 97.)

the same direction (*Fig.* 1 C). The amounts of pressure exerted at either end of the second limb of the spring are equalized by activating the second limb a little more than the first limb. In this way a row of teeth, such as four incisors, can be moved the same distance in the same direction in a row.★ (*See Figs.* 86, 88.)

The Application of Springs to Teeth.—Pressure can only be applied to a tooth at a single point using a spring. It is impossible to *grasp* a tooth with a spring. It is therefore important to see that a spring impinges on the correct point on any tooth that is to be moved. As both the spring wire and the tooth surface are hard and polished, virtually no friction exists between them so that the pressure of a spring on a tooth, even when the tooth surface slopes, is at right angles to the tooth surface at that point. The direction in which a tooth

---

★ Wild (1950) discusses the action of this spring in considerable detail.

is being pushed is, therefore, determined by the point at which the spring bears and not always by the direction of movement of the free end of the spring (*Fig.* 3).

The Type of Movement produced by Removable Appliances.—As a general rule, removable appliances tilt the teeth, producing movement of the crowns. The apices of the teeth so moved may tend to a greater or lesser extent

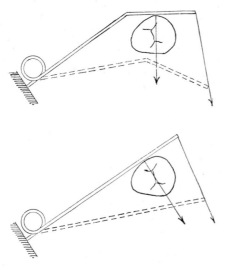

Fig. 3.—The direction in which pressure acts on a tooth does not always correspond with the direction of movement of the free end of the spring, but is determined by the point of application of the spring to the tooth.

to follow the crowns. Controlled movement of the roots of the teeth cannot easily be achieved with removable appliances, and this limitation of removable appliance technique must be borne in mind when planning treatment. A limited degree of root movement can be carried out with removable appliances in certain situations.

TWIN WIRE ARCH, ROUND ARCH, EDGEWISE ARCH

These appliances cannot be analysed into a clearly distinguishable framework or fixed part and spring or active part. A number, and in some cases all, of the teeth are banded and a bracket or attachment placed on each band.

The archwire is formed to an "ideal" or any other desired shape and is ligatured into the attachments, producing a distortion of the archwire. This distortion of the archwire gives rise to tensions which are exerted continuously on the teeth until the archwire has returned to its original shape, bringing the teeth with it. The amount of pressure required to distort these arches is high.* The arches are supported in short sections between the teeth, giving what is in effect a large series of very short stiff beam springs. A pressure of 20 g. does not produce a noticeable bending of such short sections of archwire unless the wires are very fine indeed, much finer than are used in practice.

In using such appliances as these, three factors serve to limit the action of the appliances and act as protective mechanisms to the periodontal structures:—

1. While high pressures may be used, the range of action of the arches is not great.
2. Where imbricated teeth are ligatured to the arch much pressure is dispersed through pressure of the teeth against each other.
3. The elasticity of the periodontal tissues cushions the teeth to some extent.

The basic movements that can be carried out with the arch type of appliance are:—

1. Labiolingual movement.
2. Rotation.
3. Root movement in a mesiodistal direction.
4. Depression and elevation of teeth.
5. Buccolingual and labiolingual root movement.
6. Space closure and opening.
7. The correction of arch relation by means of intermaxillary and extra-oral traction.

Labiolingual movement and rotation of incisors are particularly easily done with the Johnson twin-wire arch appliance. The two fine archwires fall into a natural curve which is approximately the curve that it is desirable

---

* It was found experimentally that a twin wire arch consisting of two 0·25-mm. wires with a span from canine to central incisor of 18 mm. from the ends of the brackets from which the arch emerged, for a pressure of 200 g. gave a deflection of less than 1 mm. A pressure of 20 g. did not produce a noticeable deflection of the arch.

that the incisors and canine teeth should occupy. When the archwires are ligatured into the brackets fixed to these teeth, pressures and tensions are brought to bear on the displaced teeth. If the irregularity is severe, as in *Fig.* 4, and the archwires have a high modulus of elasticity, and are ligatured completely into all displaced tooth brackets, very

If they are not free to move, the pressure is further dispersed against the next teeth in the arch on either side. A persistent attempt to aline incisors which are imbricated and for which no room exists or has been made in the arch will, through this tendency to spreading of the arch, produce an expansion in a forward direction and a resulting increase in overjet.

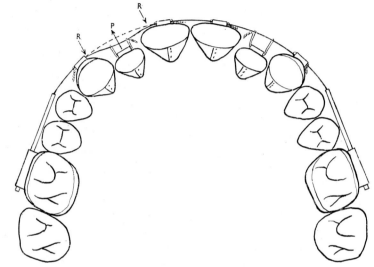

Fig. 4.—Labial movement with twin wire arch. P, Pressure on 2|; R, Reaction. The reaction is borne mainly by the adjoining teeth. The ligature on |2 has not been tightened.

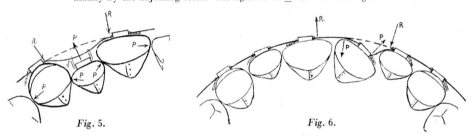

Fig. 5.   Fig. 6.

Fig. 5.—When the incisors are imbricated the full pressure, P, of the twin wire arch is not taken by the single displaced tooth. The reaction, RR, remains the same on the adjoining teeth, but the pressure, P, is dispersed against their sloping lingual surfaces, forcing them apart, and hence against the next two teeth in the row.

Fig. 6.—Rotation of incisor with twin wire arch.

severe pressures can be placed on teeth if there is space for them to move into. In *Fig.* 5, however, the lateral incisor is impacted between the canine and the central incisor, so that much of the pressure released by the twin wire arch is dispersed against the canine and central incisor, and this results in a tendency for these teeth to move apart, if they are free to do so.

The same mechanism is used to produce rotation with the twin wire arch (*Fig.* 6). A mechanical couple bears on the rotated tooth, bringing it automatically into correct alinement as the archwires return to their position of rest.

Depression and elevation of individual incisor teeth are also easily carried out with the twin

5

wire arch. Where a tooth is to be elongated it is usual only to ligature one of the archwires into the channel because it is necessary to exert a very gentle force for this particular

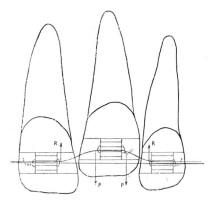

Fig. 7.—Elongation of tooth with twin wire arch. Light pressure is used; the reaction is unlikely to upset the adjoining teeth.

movement. The apical vessels and nerves are particularly susceptible to injury by excessive elongating forces (*Fig.* 7).

which result tip the tooth in a mesiodistal direction. The relative degrees of movement of the apex and the crown can be controlled by either preventing the crown from moving, in which case most movement will take place at the apex (*Fig.* 8 D), or by assisting the crown in moving, in which case most of the movement will take place at the crown and the apex will hardly move at all (*Fig.* 8 C).

Mesiodistal root movement can be effected in the buccal segments either with the "round arch" or with the edgewise arch with the use of second-order bends (*Fig.* 9). Where the arch crosses the bracket channels, it is stepped so that it crosses the channel obliquely. The arch therefore has to be twisted almost straight before it can be seated in the channel and the resulting stresses tend to tip the tooth mesiodistally. Here again, the crown tends to move in the opposite direction to the apex, and this tendency may be prevented or encouraged depending on the relative amounts of crown and root movement required. This process of tipping the teeth in the buccal segments may

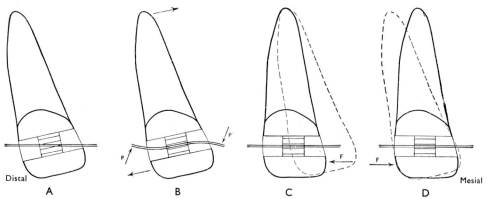

Fig. 8.—Mesiodistal root movement with the twin wire arch. A, Arch passive. B, Arch must be deformed to get into the bracket. The resulting pressures tend to move root mesially, crown distally. C, If crown is assisted by force, F, movement will be mostly at the crown. D, If crown is stabilized with force, F, movement will take place entirely at the apex.

A special property of the "arch and bracket" type of appliance is that of being able to tip the apices of the teeth in various directions. If the archwire does not run parallel to the channel in the bracket on a tooth (*Fig.* 8 A) the arch must be deformed before it can be fitted into the channel and ligatured into place (*Fig.* 8 B). The tensions in the archwire

be applied to all the teeth in a buccal segment simultaneously by fitting an arch which has a series of steps. Each step corresponds to the channel in the bracket on a tooth in the buccal segment. In order to seat the arch in the brackets, the steps must be straightened slightly and as a result a tipping force is brought to bear on every tooth in the buccal segment which is caused to tip *en masse* at the crowns or at the apices as the operator desires.

The opening and closing of spaces by mesiodistal movement of teeth or of groups of teeth can be effected with the arch type of appliance in a number of ways.

carried out with one of the round wire arch techniques or with the edgewise arch. For this purpose the archwire itself can be formed into a spring which can have an opening or a closing activity as required and the segments of teeth on either side of the space are moved as a whole, a movement that may be one of

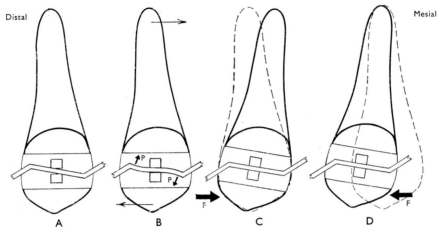

Fig. 9.—The edgewise arch—second-order bends. **A,** The passive arch crosses the bracket at an angle. **B.** The archwire is deformed in order to get it into the channel and the resulting pressures, **PP,** tend to tilt the apex mesially, the crown distally. **C,** If the crown is stabilized with a force, **F,** movement takes place at the apex. **D,** If the crown is assisted to move by force, **F,** main movement will take place at crown and not at apex.

Teeth may be moved along the archwire by simply placing a wire ligature around the bracket on the tooth to be moved and ligating the tooth to a convenient anchorage point mesially or distally. By a series of small adjustments of the ligature the tooth can be gradually drawn in the direction required. By using a fine elastic ligature or an elastic band, or by placing a small length of expanded coil spring on the archwire between a wire ligature and the bracket attached to the tooth, a longer range of action can be given to the appliance, with a corresponding increase in time between visits for adjustments. A coil spring placed on an archwire between two teeth can be used to move the teeth apart.

Mesiodistal movements such as these can be effected with twin wire arches, plain round wire arches, or with the edgewise arch. Movements of space closure or opening involving the movement of the complete groups of teeth on either side of the space are usually

opening or of closing as required. At all times the axial inclination of the teeth is controlled by the fitting of the archwire in the slot in the bracket, although in some techniques, such as that advocated by Begg (1965), the tilting of the teeth is controlled by auxiliary springs fitted in addition to the archwire and the teeth can be tipped freely about their point of attachment to the archwire in any direction.

A further root movement that may be performed with the edgewise arch is bucco- or labiolingual movement of the apices of the teeth by twisting or torquing the arch (*Fig.* 10). The arch wire fits very accurately into the brackets on the bands and the twist in the arch is transformed into a tipping in a labiolingual direction of front teeth or in a buccolingual direction of the cheek teeth.

As already mentioned, all these appliances give rise to complicated anchorage problems. The reactions from the stressed sections of the

7

arches are applied directly to the adjoining teeth and, on account of the continuity of the dental arch, to the teeth immediately beyond. The effect of these forces of reaction has to be carefully assessed and appropriate steps taken to make sure that no unwanted tooth movements take place.

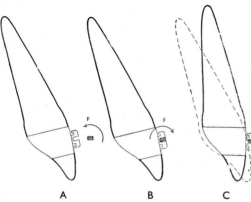

Fig. 10.—Torque force applied to an incisor using the edgewise arch for labial root movement. A, The arch must be twisted with a force, F, to aline it with the channel in the bracket and permit insertion. B, The arch then exerts force, F, tipping the apex of the tooth labially. The amount of pressure exerted on the labial plate of bone is difficult to assess clinically. C, Movement produced by torque force.

Intermaxillary and extra-oral traction are frequently used with all these appliances for the purpose of correcting arch relationships and for securing adequate anchorage in some cases. There is an extensive literature dealing with these fixed appliances, and it is impossible here to do more than indicate the elementary principles of their action. The reader is referred to more extensive works which give the many refinements that are incorporated in the appliances in the treatment of various types of case.

It would be naïve to assume that in practice a tooth will move in response to the arch type of appliance exactly as planned according to the mechanical action of the section of arch applied to it. These appliances introduce such a complexity of pressures and reactions into the dental arch that it is sometimes difficult or impossible to assess exactly how much pressure is being applied at any one spot. Furthermore, root form influences the movement

of the teeth mechanically and the small alterations in occlusal relation and the relation of the teeth in the same arch affects the distribution of stress from day to day. Lastly, the alveolar bone is a living tissue and it does not always react in a purely mechanical way to mechanical stresses.

When an arch type of appliance has been planned and put into position, it must be carefully watched and accurate assessments made of changes that occur and particular care taken that relative movements are not mistaken for the precise movements that are the objectives aimed at.

FUNCTIONAL APPLIANCES

Functional appliances are appliances which make use of the pressures which exist in and about the oral cavity either by using these pressures actively through the medium of the appliance to exert pressures upon the teeth or by inhibiting muscular or soft tissue pressures, either normal or abnormal, which are being exerted upon the teeth, thus allowing other factors such as eruption or opposing pressures to produce tooth movement.

Functional appliances, acting as they do by harnessing existing functional stresses, do not as a rule have active elements incorporated in them. Sometimes, however, this rule is not followed and active springs or archwires, screens, or resilient pads are incorporated in the appliance in order to bestow greater versatility, but such elaborations should be carefully controlled as they may make the resulting appliance too complicated.

Well-known functional appliances are the anterior bite plane, the inclined plane, and the oral screen which are of simple construction and produce well defined changes in the distribution of stresses in the masticatory apparatus. The Andresen appliance and the Function Corrector are more complicated in design and also in their modes of action. The design, construction, and uses of all these appliances are discussed in greater detail in Chapter XI.

TRACTION WITH ELASTIC BANDS

In appliances using traction, energy is stored in elastic bands under tension. This energy is applied to single teeth by means of a band attached to the tooth carrying a hook or to a group of teeth through the medium of fixed or removable appliances. The line of action of a force applied in this way is along the line of the elastic band. Elastic traction may be used as intramaxillary traction, intermaxillary traction, or extra-oral traction. In each instance the amount of pressure exerted on the tooth or teeth is regulated by the length of the elastic used and the amount of extension of the elastic. Using elastic traction it is possible to apply a very heavy pressure over a long range of action. It is important, therefore, when applying elastic traction to see that the heaviest pressure used is related to the number of teeth being moved, and, where single or small numbers of teeth are being moved, not to apply an excessive pressure.

SCREW APPLIANCES

The expansion screw consists essentially of a screw which fits into an internally threaded sleeve. The sleeve is embedded in one part of the appliance and the head of the screw in the other. Turning the screw causes the two sections of the appliance to move apart. The screw appliance can indeed be used in this simple form, and the screw can be operated by rotating the two parts of the appliance with respect to each other through a complete revolution. It is possible to use a screw in an even simpler form, for small individual tooth movements, by driving a plain brass machine screw through the baseplate opposite the tooth which it is required to move. Adjustments are made at the usual intervals with a small screwdriver. (Hallett, 1952.)

Most screws, however, are made with several useful refinements. A guide rod or two guide rods are provided to ensure that the two parts of the appliance move apart in a strictly parallel fashion without rocking or twisting. A friction device may be provided to stiffen the action of the screw so that it can only be turned by means of a key or pin.

The expansion screw designed by J. H. Badcock (1911), and widely known as the Badcock screw, consists of a robustly designed screw and sleeve which give the device its main strength. The guide rod and its sleeve are of lighter construction and serve to prevent the two parts of the appliance from rotating with respect to each other. The screw has a square nut which is turned by means of a wrench. The faces of the nut are numbered. (*Fig.* 11.)

The Glenross screw employs two guides and a central, screwed rod. This rod has a spherical nut in the middle and both ends of the rod are threaded, one end with a right- and the other with a left-hand thread. Bending and other stresses not actually concerned with the expansion are shared about equally between the screw and the two guide rods. The screw is turned by means of a pin which is inserted into one of four holes situated equidistantly around the circumference of the nut. Quarter turns may thus be given. The whole screw is flat and compact. (*Fig.* 12.)

Screws of different design but operating on the same principle as those already mentioned are produced in different countries. Certain screws incorporate a spring so that when the screw is opened, the appliance can be compressed against the spring. Energy is then stored in the spring inside the screw. In conventional screws there is no spring.

The screw or split plate, using conventional screws, is a rigid appliance. When a screw appliance is opened up and pushed into place, immediate movement of the teeth must occur. The amount of movements that result from a single adjustment of the screw is very small, that is to say the range of action of the appliance is very small. The action of the rigid screw plate depends on the fact that there is a slight normal degree of mobility of the teeth owing to a slight elasticity of the periodontal tissues—firstly the periodontal membrane and probably also the periodontal bone. It is in this elastic tissue that the energy is stored which, acting on the alveolar bone, produces the processes of resorption and deposition of bone that lead to re-formation of the socket about the tooth root, which is already in its new position. In practice, before this process of re-formation of the socket can be completed, the tooth is moved again by a

9

further adjustment of the screw, and so an extensive tooth movement can gradually be carried out.

Adjustment of the Screw.—The amount of expansion produced by a quarter, a half, or rate at which the screw should be turned will depend on the rate at which the periodontal tissues react to the pressure exerted on them, and this reaction is the best guide to the operation of screws. Normally the screw is

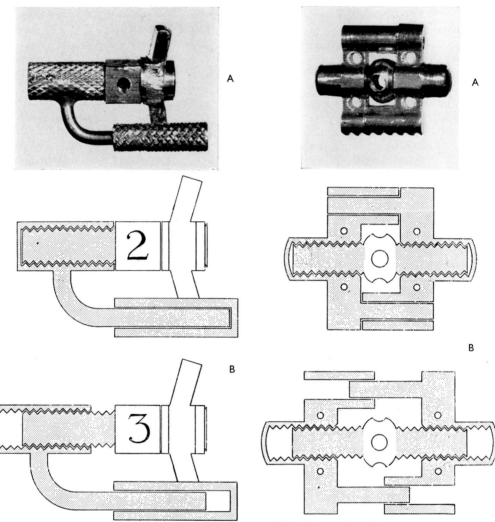

Fig. 11.—**A**, The Badcock expansion screw. **B**, The action of the Badcock screw: above, closed; below, partially opened. (*By kind permission of the Amalgamated Dental Co. Ltd., London.*)

Fig. 12.—**A**, The Glenross expansion screw. This is the small size which measures 12 × 9·5 mm. **B**, The action of the Glenross screw: above, closed; below, partially opened. (*By kind permission of Glenross Ltd., London.*)

one full turn of a screw can be determined by means of callipers or a micrometer. The information so obtained is of interest but is not essential to clinical use of screws. The given one-quarter of a turn at a time and the rate of tooth movement is regulated by the frequency with which this adjustment is made. The patient can tell at once when the appliance

10

has been adjusted, by the sensation of stiffness and tension in the periodontal membrane.

If subsequent adjustments are made at too short intervals and, in consequence, expansion is attempted too rapidly, one of two effects results: either the patient complains of the increasing pressure and discomfort and leaves the appliance out; or else the appliance cannot be fully seated in position in the mouth and gradually creeps out of position up the sloping surfaces of the teeth and eventually ceases to fit altogether.

To a great extent, therefore, screw appliances are self-limiting in their action. This feature, and the fact that adjustment of the screw can usually be left to the patient, makes the screw type of appliance extremely useful in those cases where the patient, for one reason or another, can only be seen at comparatively long intervals of time.

Screw pressure can be used for the movement of large numbers of teeth, as for instance in expansion, or for the movement of individual teeth or teeth in small groups. The use of screw pressure to produce a wide variety of tooth movements is demonstrated by Schwarz, 1956. Appliances using screw pressure are often referred to as "Schwarz appliances".

ANCHORAGE

The dispersal of the reaction from the pressure exerted by an orthodontic appliance must be so arranged that other useful work is done or so that at least no untoward effects take place. Orthodontic appliances, being attached to teeth, tend through the reaction to disturb anchorage teeth as an undesirable side-effect. In certain instances these ill effects can be avoided if the appliance is so constructed that equal and opposite pressures are exerted on similar teeth or groups of teeth in order to move them equal or proportional amounts in opposite directions. In such instances the action and reaction are both producing required tooth movement. (*See Figs.* 115, 131, 132.) Where a single tooth, or a group of teeth, is to be moved in one direction only, care must be taken to ensure that the reaction does not also produce tooth movement.

Anchorage may be obtained from three sources:—

1. Within the same dental arch in which tooth movements are being carried out.

2. By intermaxillary traction to the opposing dental arch.

3. From outside the mouth altogether by means of occipital or cervical anchorage.

Anchorage within the same arch is achieved by arranging the appliance so that as many teeth as possible are incorporated in the anchorage section of the appliance and attempting to move as few teeth as possible at a time.

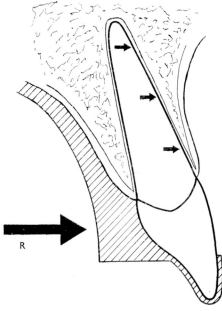

Fig. 13.—"Stationary anchorage". The incisor that is capped cannot tip forward at the crown and hence the reaction, R, is distributed evenly along the labial wall of the socket, so reducing the pressure in terms of grammes per square millimetre of bone area. It is necessary to see that the thickness of baseplate material on the lingual surface of the upper incisors does not interfere with the occlusion. In the case above an anterior biteplate is being used. (*See Fig.* 121, p. 79.)

In this way the anchorage teeth will outnumber the teeth to be moved and the pressure in terms of grammes per square millimetre of root area of the anchorage will be so low that disturbance of these teeth will not easily take place.

11

In arranging anchorage, four important factors must be borne in mind:—

1. The natural tendency for tooth movement in the arch.
2. Lip posture and function.
3. Occlusal interlock.
4. The pressure required to move teeth.

The operation of these factors and their influence on tooth movement must be carefully assessed in any given case when treatment is being planned. The teeth in the buccal segments, particularly the molars, have a tendency to move forward as part of the developmental process of the occlusion. If these teeth are used as anchorage to resist a reaction in a forward direction, this tendency to forward movement may be increased— that is to say, movement of anchorage teeth may take place. Conversely, the tendency of the teeth in the buccal segments to forward movements makes them more resistant to a reaction in a backward direction.

Faulty lip and tongue posture may lead to reduction in the stability of the position of the incisor teeth and make it easy for them to be proclined by the reaction of an appliance if they are used as part of the anchorage. Loss of occlusal interlock which occurs if bite planes are used may lead to instability in one or other arch and movement of anchor teeth under quite small pressures.

The pressure required to move teeth falls between a minimum below which activation of the surrounding bone does not occur at all, and a maximum above which pain and damage to the tooth and periodontal tissues will occur. If the pressure per tooth in the anchorage segment can be kept below the minimum required to produce tooth movement, no movement of anchorage should take place.

In certain instances it is possible to increase the resistance of anchor teeth to movement by locking them so that they cannot tilt. This applies exclusively to incisors where removable appliances are concerned, but the principle is often applied to the teeth in the buccal segments in fixed appliance treatment. Teeth are more resistant to bodily movement than they are to tilting, and this bodily movement takes longer to effect than a tilting movement. If the upper incisors are locked into the plate by capping their incisal edges (*Fig.* 13 and *Fig.* 121, p. 79), they are very resistant to forward movement and their value as anchorage teeth may be thus very much increased.

12

CHAPTER II

THE DESIGN OF REMOVABLE APPLIANCES

THE design of a removable appliance must begin with a detailed plan of the tooth movements that are to be carried out in the course of the treatment of the case under consideration. It should also be foreseen in considerable detail at this stage how many appliances are going to be used and what their construction is likely to be. If the treatment plan is at all of a complicated nature, involving a number of different tooth movements in different directions, it is important to consider carefully how many movements can be carried out with one appliance alone and if necessary to break down the treatment plan into a series of simple tooth movements using a separate appliance for each. Many failures of treatment and consequent condemnation of the removable appliance technique result from misguided attempts to simplify and shorten treatment by trying to move too many teeth all in different directions using a multiplicity of springs on one appliance. This criticism does not refer to the movement of considerable numbers of teeth in one direction such as occurs, for instance, as a result of intermaxillary traction. Here the appliance and form of pressure applied are essentially simple and straightforward.

When a large number of different movements is attempted by means of a number of springs on a single appliance, two distinct difficulties usually arise: firstly, too few teeth are left for anchorage purposes and for clasping to retain the appliance; and, secondly, the patient may be faced with a too complicated appliance to insert. He may not be able to compress all the springs simultaneously to enable him to put the appliance in position. It is very much better to use a number of appliances for successive movements, this method having the great advantage that after a movement is completed the appliance can be used as a retainer until the next appliance

is ready for insertion, so avoiding relapse and unwanted tooth movement while the new appliance is under construction.

When designing an appliance, a great many considerations have to be balanced against one another, and, while these factors need to be taken individually, no single one need always dominate the entire process; they all react upon each other, and in different cases different considerations will have different degrees of importance. A removable appliance should be designed to produce the desired tooth movements without the need for constant adjustment—that is to say, all springs should continue to act if possible over the whole distance that teeth require to be moved, and at the same time appliances should interfere as little as possible with the everyday activities of the patient and in particular with the maintenance of an adequate degree of oral cleanliness. These requirements necessitate a detailed consideration of tooth movements required, design of springs, anchorage, clasping of the appliance, design of baseplate, comfort of the patient, and the patient's capacity to manage an orthodontic appliance.

TOOTH MOVEMENTS

For the purposes of discussing appliance design, tooth movements may conveniently be considered as falling into the following categories: labio- and bucco-lingual movement; mesiodistal movement; rotation; and root movement. If the treatment plan is broken down into a succession of such movements the simplest means of performing each movement or set of movements can be determined. While labio- and bucco-lingual, mesiodistal, and rotation and root movements refer to the movement of individual teeth, expansion is simply a buccal or labial movement of an entire segment, and intermaxillary traction is usually arranged to produce movement of a number of teeth mesially or distally in the buccal segments and labially or lingually in the labial segments.

THE DESIGN OF SPRINGS

With a view to avoiding the need of frequent adjustments, springs should be made as a rule with a range of action as long or slightly longer than the distance over which the tooth is to be moved. There are obvious advantages in thick wires for springs, in that they will be less likely to damage at the hands of the patient and less likely to become displaced from their point of application to the tooth under conditions found in the mouth; but such springs are bound to have a short range of action and require frequent adjustment. The range of action of thick springs may be increased by increasing the length of the spring, and this would be the most desirable way of procuring springs with a long range of action. There are, unfortunately, definite limits to the length of finger springs imposed by the dimensions of the dental arches and the depth of the buccal and lingual sulci, and these dimensions limit the length of springs to such an extent that thick springs, that is to say of 0·7 mm. thickness or larger, such as can be placed on orthodontic appliances, usually have a very short useful range of action. Thick springs have, however, definite uses and advantages in certain circumstances, and the short range of action that goes with them is accepted as a necessary evil and short intervals between visits are arranged accordingly.

The range of action of springs is usually lengthened by making them of thinner wire and also by putting a coil or a number of coils at the point of attachment of the spring. The use of thinner wire for springs makes it necessary to adopt certain measures to ensure that the spring will act efficiently, because springs made of thin wires are not self-supporting and are liable to damage and displacement in the mouth and require to be guided and protected to ensure their efficient activity.

Simplicity in spring design is very much to be desired. The straightforward cantilever spring, fixed at one end and movable at the other, can be constructed in a wide range of gauges and lengths of wire and is adaptable to a great variety of situations. This type of spring has the further advantages that its mode of action is clear and obvious and patients find it easy to compress and hold in position while inserting the appliance. In some instances this spring is almost completely automatic and needs little attention from the patient (*see Figs.* 98, 101).

When planning the layout of springs it is necessary to visualize the path of movement of the free end of the spring and to make this correspond if possible with the desired path of movement of the tooth to be moved. Only in this way will the greatest efficiency of the spring be developed. At the same time the point of application of the spring to the tooth must be observed because, as mentioned earlier, the effective pressure on a tooth is at right angles to the tangent at the point of application of the spring, there being no friction, for practical purposes, between a spring and the hard surface of the tooth. While it is important to place the point of attachment of the spring at a point which will make the movement of the free end correspond with the desired movement of the tooth, this ideal cannot always be achieved, and it is then necessary to adjust the point of application of the spring to the tooth with some care. It is also necessary to look out for any alteration in the point of application of the spring to the tooth that may result from tooth movement and to see that the spring remains applied to the correct spot on the tooth.

There are two broad groups of finger springs: The self-supporting springs of 0·7 mm. thickness or heavier; and the guided and protected springs of 0·5 mm. thickness or lighter. Springs of 0·6-mm. wire may come into one class or the other depending on the details of their design. Coil springs fall into a special and distinct category.

The Self-supporting Springs.—These are, as their name suggests, capable of standing up of their own accord to the interference of the soft tissues of the mouth during speech and mastication without suffering

14

damage and do not injure the soft tissues which lie against them. At the same time they are sufficiently flexible to enjoy a small but useful range of action (*see Figs.* 101, 112, 116). These springs are used in situations in which there is not enough space to permit the use of a heavy wire as framework and a fine wire as spring, or where this latter combination is not adaptable to produce the kind of movement required. The wire used for a spring of this type must combine in itself sufficient rigidity to avoid distortion by the pressures encountered in the mouth and to maintain its point of application to the tooth and sufficient elasticity to be effective as a spring. These qualities are found in their best proportion in wires of 0·7 mm. and 0·6 mm. gauge. It will be noted that in most of these springs the introduction of a coil half-way along the spring has the effect of giving the spring a longer range of action at its operating end without affecting the rigidity of the spring as a whole which is determined by the stiff proximal limb.

Protected and Guided Springs.—These springs are distinguished by being made of a thin wire, that is 0·5 mm. thick or smaller, and by having one or more coils at their point of attachment. These characteristics give the springs a long range of action but make them also flexible in a plane at right angles to the plane in which they are desired to operate. The springs are, therefore, liable to become displaced when in action owing to the fact that they cannot grasp the tooth but can only impinge on the hard, smooth, enamel surface. If this surface happens to be even only slightly inclined to the plane of action of a spring of this kind, and not at right angles to it, the spring will tend to slip along the surface then afforded. This of course will mean that the point of application of the spring will become different from that which was intended and the wrong effect may result, or the spring fail to act efficiently.

There are various ways in which a fine spring may be kept under control and made to act precisely on a tooth. The standard finger spring of 0·5-mm. wire, usually about 20 mm. long with one coil of 3–4 mm. diameter,

can be controlled by means of a wire or guide overlying it (*Figs.* 14, 85, 95, 113, 115). A single wire or elongated loop of wire is as a rule sufficient, and if the reaction of the spring against the tooth urges the spring against the guide wire, very adequate control of the spring can be achieved. If it is anticipated that a spring of this kind will be difficult to control for any reason, a double guide wire, one above and one below (*Fig.* 14 C), may be made.

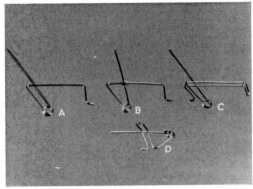

Fig. 14.—A, Spring with guide; B, Spring with guide and link; C, Spring with double guide; D, Incisor spring with guide.

Alternatively, the spring may be linked to the guide wire by a small link of fine hard wire (*Fig.* 15). This most effectively limits the unwanted vertical movement of the spring.

A further method of protecting and guiding a spring of fine gauge wire is to box it in under the baseplate of removable appliances (*Fig.* 16). This is sometimes the only feasible method, but it has few advantages and many disadvantages. The cavity beneath the plate is an ideal site for the collection of debris and the gingival tissue in some instances will hypertrophy into the space and interfere with and become injured by the spring. The spring cannot be provided with a really smooth surface to run against. The spring may be displaced permanently away from the baseplate by carelessness on the part of the patient and may be difficult to adjust back into position. It is impossible to tie a spring against a plate to prevent displacement of the spring along a sloping tooth surface. On

15

the other hand, when a baseplate is weak at the point where a spring is placed, boxing in the spring may make the plate stronger at this point. When this is done a guide wire as well will ensure the smooth running of the spring (*see Fig.* 128).

As a general rule guide wires should be placed as near to the moving end of the spring as possible in order to achieve the greatest possible degree of control over the movement of the spring. Guide wires should hold the spring down to the point at which pressure is to be put upon the tooth. The spring and

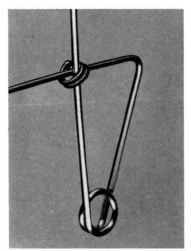

Fig. 15.—A link will hold a spring wire against the guide wire. Link is made of 0·3-mm. wire, wound around twice, cut off, and loosened sufficiently by running a probe through it.

guide wire must be made so as to lie as flatly as possible against the palate or gingival tissue in the lower jaw, or neatly in the buccal or labial sulcus as the case may be.

The finer springs, of 0·35 mm. and 0·3 mm. thickness (*see Figs.* 90, 101, 107), are coiled around and supported from the outset on a framework or arch of heavy wire. These springs are fairly short in the limb and derive their elasticity from the three or four coils that are wound around the supporting arch. The spring wire is fine and flexible in every direction, but is made more stable by returning the free end to the archwire and winding the wire around the arch once or twice. A spring

so constructed will thus have a V or U shape which is very rigid and reduces the movement of the spring to a single plane which is the desired plane of action. This kind of spring has a long range of action in relation to its length and for this reason the free end traces

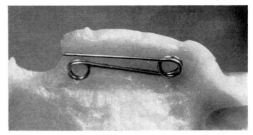

Fig. 16.—Spring guided by boxing under baseplate. Further control of this spring may be achieved by bending the free end at right angles, so forming an arm which will run beneath the acrylic plane and prevent the free end of the spring from rising above the level of the plane.

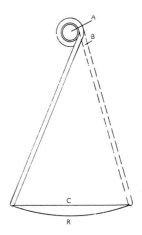

Fig. 17.—A, Foundation arch. B, Auxiliary spring. R, Path of free end of spring. C, Chord of arc described by free end of spring. When the range of action of a spring is long in relation to the length of the arm of the spring, the free end of the spring moves in a marked curve. The effective line of action of the spring is the chord of this arc, but the effects of the changing direction of movement of the free end of the spring should be anticipated.

a path which is markedly curved. For practical purposes, however, the effective line of action of the free end of the spring is the chord of the arc so traced (*Fig.* 17). As this kind of spring is frequently used to produce proclination and retroclination of the incisor

16

teeth, the movement of the spring will in fact correspond with the tooth movement that takes place.

Springs: their Range and Pressure.—The amount of pressure that is exerted by a spring, when activated and the appliance placed in the

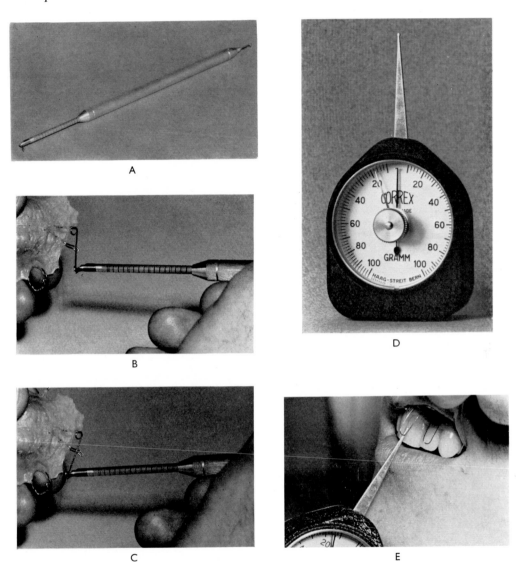

Fig. 18.—The use of a pressure gauge. A, A plunger type of pressure gauge which can be used to push at one end and pull at the other. The plunger rod is graduated. B, C, Testing the pressure of a finger spring. The spring is depressed by the amount that is used when the appliance is placed in the mouth and the pressure read from the calibrations on the gauge. D, The "Correx" pressure gauge. Pressure at either side of the tip of the lever produces a deflection of the needle on the dial of the instrument. The amount of the dial reading is recorded by the second needle attached to the knurled button placed in the glass cover. E, Using the "Correx" gauge to measure the pressure of an apron spring. The liver is slipped under the spring which is then lifted away from the tooth. The pressure exerted by the spring is recorded on the dial of the gauge. This is a very convenient and accurate gauge. The diameter of the dial is 3·5 cm. (Obtainable from Hawley, Russell & Baker Limited, Leighton House, 35 Darkes Lane, Potters Bar, Herts.)

mouth, can be simply determined by the use of an orthodontic pressure gauge which is designed so that any spring can be lifted a little from its point of application using the pressure gauge and the amount of force required to displace the spring is indicated by the gauge.

Alternatively, the spring may be checked on the bench by deflecting the spring to the amount used in the mouth, by means of the pressure gauge, and noting the pressure required. (*Fig.* 18.)

Orthodontic appliances in use should be checked in this way from time to time, but it will be found that the same kinds of springs are used repeatedly in different situations and familiarity with their use and observation of the reaction of the tissues to the action of the appliance will be found a satisfactory guide to the correct degree of activity of the springs. As a further aid to the use of such springs and appliances *Table I* gives the construction of a

pressure exerted by the spring (*see Figs.* 85, 94, 96). It is important, of course, to use every other available tooth in the arch as anchorage when moving even one or two teeth by means of a spring. Only in this way is it possible to ensure that the required tooth is moved with minimal disturbance of anchorage teeth.

Anchorage problems have to be given more careful consideration when large or multi-rooted teeth are being moved or when several teeth are to be moved in the same direction. When large teeth such as upper canines or molars are to be moved, it is quite legitimate to exert rather greater pressures upon them than the minimal 20 g. Again, when a number of teeth are being moved in the same direction the individual pressures on these teeth may add up to quite a large total with a correspondingly large reaction to be dispersed. If in these circumstances the number of anchorage teeth is inadequate or the teeth have any natural tendency to move in the

Table I.—TABLE OF PRESSURES OF SPRINGS

SPRING TYPE	LENGTH (mm.)	THICKNESS (mm.)	No. OF COILS	INNER DIAMETER OF COILS (mm.)	DEFLECTION FOR 20 G. PRESSURE (mm.)
Apron (*Fig.* 101)	12	0·3	4	1·0	9·0
Finger (*Fig.* 85)	18	0·5	1	2·5	3·0
Self-supporting	10	0·7	1	3·5	0·3
(*Fig.* 116)	15	0·7	1	4·0	0·6

number of typical springs, and the amount of deflection produced by a pressure of 20 g. is shown.

THE PLANNING OF ANCHORAGE

Although the number of teeth to be moved will dictate the minimum amount of anchorage required, it is much better to be on the safe side and achieve as much anchorage as possible when considering the movement of any given tooth or group of teeth.

The movement of single teeth does not as a rule raise any great anchorage problem. All the other teeth in the same arch, and in the maxilla, the support given to the baseplate by its contact with the palate, provide adequate resistance to the reaction of the

same direction as the reaction, there may be movement of anchorage teeth instead of the teeth requiring to be moved.

This kind of problem is exemplified in the retraction of the teeth in the anterior segment of the upper arch. The teeth in the buccal segments have a tendency to move forward as a part of the developmental process of the occlusion. If the teeth in the buccal segments are used as anchorage to resist a distal pressure, the reaction to which will of course be in a forward direction, this reaction will tend to bring forward the teeth in the buccal segments even more rapidly, so taking up space anteriorly.

The upper canines are large-rooted teeth which require a considerable time for their movement and a considerable pressure can be exerted on them without ill effects. For these reasons, the retraction of upper canines into the space created by the extraction of the first premolars must be performed with care if the teeth in the upper buccal segments are used as anchorage for this movement. Unless precautions are taken to avoid it, there is a distinct tendency for the buccal segments to move forward as well as, or instead of, the canines moving backward. This tendency may be reduced or eliminated entirely by constructing the baseplate of the appliance so that it impinges on every tooth in the arch (*Fig.* 118). This reaction is, therefore, distributed over every tooth and over the anterior surface of the palate, so achieving the maximum possible anchorage. At the same time the pressure put upon the canines should not be allowed to become excessive, as this will tend to raise the pressure per unit of anchorage to a level which may produce movement of anchorage teeth.

The same problem arises in connexion with the retraction of the upper incisor segment in a lingual direction using the teeth in the buccal segments as anchorage. In this situation factors that must be taken into account are the additional resistance that may need to be overcome owing to the pressure of the lower lip behind the upper incisors, the fact that only the teeth in the buccal segments are available as anchorage, and the tendency to come forward spontaneously that these teeth usually show.

It is sometimes suggested that it is not feasible to retract the upper incisor segment using only the buccal segments as anchorage because of the tendency of the buccal segments to come forward.

It is true that if an excessive pressure is exerted on the teeth in the labial segment, the reaction to this pressure may bring the buccal segments forward. This untoward effect may be avoided by eschewing the use of high pressures and by making use of the anchorage of the buccal segments to the best advantage in the following ways. Firstly, every available tooth must be used—that is to say, the baseplate must be taken distally to the last tooth in the arch. Secondly, the

baseplate must fit accurately and be clasped firmly; this has the effect of preventing the buccal segments from approximating each other in a lateral direction, and if this is made impossible, they will be less likely to come forward because if they are to come forward they must needs come on to a narrower part of the alveolar arch and must therefore come nearer to each other in a lateral direction. Thirdly, the pressure exerted on the teeth to be moved should be kept down to a level at which the reaction will be unlikely to disturb the anchorage teeth. This will mean the use of a sensitive type of spring having a long range of action and if necessary moving only two teeth at a time. The individual type of spring shown in *Figs.* 101, 104 is most useful for this purpose as it is possible to vary the pressure on individual teeth and to vary the point of application of the spring on each tooth.

The tendency to forward movement of the buccal segments also raises problems in the lower arch when this arch is used as anchorage for the application of intermaxillary traction to the teeth in the upper arch. In certain cases forward movement of the teeth in the lower buccal segments is anticipated and desired, but in other cases this effect definitely is not required, and, should it occur as a result of intermaxillary traction, it may at a later date lead to a crowding together of the teeth in the labial segment, resulting in imbrication of the incisors and overlapping of the canines over the lateral incisors.

Where this effect is definitely to be avoided and the lower arch must yet be used for anchorage purposes, certain precautions should be taken. Firstly, all possible teeth should be incorporated for anchorage purposes. Secondly, the whole dental arch should be locked together in continuity as closely as possible. Thirdly, the principle of "stationary anchorage" should be used. Fourthly, the total force applied should be kept as low as possible.

The removable lower traction plate (*see Fig.* 140) is designed to incorporate these features. All the teeth in front of and including the first permanent molars are embraced in the anchorage segment. If the second molar can be included as anchorage by means of

19

wire running distally to it, this should be done. The provision of a labial bow which touches the incisors and canines near to their incisal edges has a double effect. The incisors are converted into sources of "stationary anchorage" and the canines are kept in the line of the arch, so preventing their riding out over the labial surfaces of the lateral incisors. The arch as a whole is therefore protected at a weak spot where a break is liable to occur. It then only remains to see that the elastic tension applied to the anchorage so provided is kept down to a safe level.

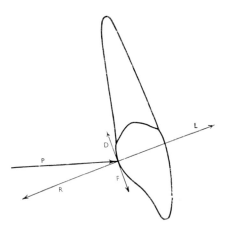

Fig. 19.—A spring exerting a pressure P on the lingual aspect of an upper incisor impinges on a sloping, frictionless surface. The effects of this force are to produce a force L at right angles to the surface impinged on, equal to the resolved part of the force P in this direction, tending to move the tooth labially; a force F parallel to the surface impinged on, equal to the resolved part of the pressure P in this direction which tends to displace the appliance downwards. The reaction R to the force L tends also to displace the appliance in a downward and backward direction. In practice the appliance is the less movable element in the pressure system, being fixed to anchorage, and the force L proclines the tooth and the reaction D to the force F tends to produce a depressing effect on the tooth.

THE DISPOSITION OF CLASPS

The selection of teeth for clasping purposes should receive some attention, and particularly so when there are not many teeth available for this purpose. Clasps should of course be placed so as to resist to the best advantage the forces tending to displace the appliance. Not all orthodontic forces tend

to displace appliances; it is those appliances that exert a force which possesses a component which acts in a vertical direction tending thereby to lift the appliance that are most likely to displace it. It is necessary, therefore, in siting clasps to consider how much tendency there is for the appliance to lift or displace and to arrange clasps accordingly. It is unnecessary to over-clasp an appliance as this represents a failure to appreciate design problems, and leads to unnecessary laboratory work.

The consideration of spring design and action will lead to a decision as to whether any springs have a vertical component of force or not. For instance, the spring in Fig. 85 acting on the sloping lingual surface of the upper incisor will have resolved parts in two directions at right angles to each other (Fig. 19). The upward component will exert a depressing force on the tooth and there will be a downward reaction of equal and opposite amount which will tend to displace the appliance. This displacing effect can be best resisted by keeping the clasps as far forward as possible. Clasps farther back do not resist the displacing force so well, as a leverage is exerted on them, the displacing force having a mechanical advantage over the clasps, and this is the greater the farther back the clasps are placed. It is always to be remembered in this connexion, however, that a clasp on a more claspable tooth farther back may be more effective than a clasp on a less claspable tooth farther forward.

The same problem arises in the lower arch where proclination of the incisors is being undertaken. The sloping lingual surfaces of the incisors give rise to a vertical reaction which has a pronounced tendency to lift up the appliance anteriorly. This effect is resisted by clasping the appliance as far forward as possible (see Fig. 90).

On the other hand, appliances used for intermaxillary and extra-oral traction, while needing to be clasped liberally to ensure overall stability, do not need to be clasped extremely tightly by each individual clasp. The pressures exerted by intermaxillary and extra-oral elastics are almost in the plane of the dental arches and in fact do not have much vertical component at all (*see Figs.* 146, 147). It is often found that patients wearing these appliances can retain them perfectly effectively with minimum clasping effort.

Appliances used for buccal and lingual movement of the cheek teeth and for lingual movement of the incisor teeth have to contend, on the whole, with reactions that are almost horizontal and there is little displacing effect. It is, therefore, as a rule sufficient where anchorage considerations permit to use a clasp on either side, arranged usually at diametrically opposite points on the arch in order to minimize rocking of the appliance (*Fig.* 96). If clasps are only placed on corresponding opposite points of the appliance in the same transverse plane, there may be a tendency for the appliance to rock anteroposteriorly.

Lower appliances are to some extent more easily retained than upper, because if the teeth are well erupted the lingual inclination of the teeth automatically tends to retain the appliance. This effect cannot always be relied on, especially in the younger patient, and great care should be given to the fit and adjustment of clasps on lower appliances.

BASEPLATE DESIGN

The baseplate has the functions of acting as a support for the springs which exert pressure on the teeth and of distributing the reaction of these springs to the anchorage. In certain types of appliance the baseplate is modified to form an active part of the appliance in the shape of biting and guiding planes. The design and construction of the baseplate can materially affect the efficiency of an appliance and the comfort of the patient and hence his willingness to undergo treatment.

Baseplates frequently require to be extended for the purposes of gaining anchorage and stability against rocking anteroposteriorly and also in order to enclose and secure the tags of clasps, arches, and auxiliary springs, but they should not at the same time be made excessively thick. As a general rule, the upper baseplate need be no thicker than a single thickness of wax. The lower baseplate, as will be explained shortly, requires different treatment.

The wider the arch over which a baseplate is spread, the less likely is the plate to rock. Rocking of a plate is a most undesirable defect as it leads to inaccuracy in the application of springs to the teeth. In the upper arch, for instance (*see Fig.* 100), it is advantageous to carry the baseplate distally as far as possible along the dental arch and distal to the last tooth in the arch. This has the double effect of reducing the tendency of the plate to rock anteroposteriorly and it also increases the anchorage to reactions acting in a forward direction. It is not necessary to extend the plate distally in the midline, but it is better to cut it away as much as possible in the midline in order to expose an adequate area of the palate to the natural friction of the tongue during speech and mastication.

It has been already suggested that springs which run on guide wires work more smoothly and are easier to adjust than those which are boxed in by the baseplate. The adjustment of the former type of spring is greatly facilitated by designing the baseplate where necessary with triangular windows within which the springs operate. It is important to see that in fact these windows are adequate and cover the entire range of action of the spring. There is little risk of weakening the baseplate if the appliance is well proportioned, of correct thickness, and the springs and guide wires are all in one piece of wire (*see Fig.* 119).

It is a useful feature to finish off all tags by turning the end down at right angles and cutting off at a length of $1\frac{1}{2}$–2 mm. This method of finishing tags is best for all clasps, bows, and springs, and has the advantage that the tag is supported away from the plaster model and a definite thickness of baseplate material flows under and around the tag. It is not necessary to make tags zig-zag wildly through the baseplate. Clasp tags going in pairs, or any wire both ends of which are embedded in the plate, need hardly be bent in a lateral direction at all. If only one end of a wire is embedded in the plate and there is any risk of its rotating, the tag may be bent at a right angle or a near right angle in a lateral direction which will obviate the possibility of rotation without making the tag unnecessarily complicated.

21

If tags are bent down and supported as described, it is only necessary to cover them with a single thickness of wax, thickening the baseplate only over the tag and not all over the available area of the baseplate (*Fig.* 20). Too often does it occur that a massive baseplate is produced with tags of clasps, arches, and auxiliary springs lying barely in the palatal surface of the plate. Such tags are very liable to come out of the plate altogether.

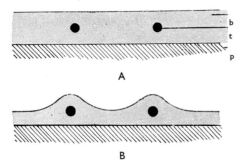

Fig. 20.—A, The plate should not be thickened uniformly all over the palate (p, palate; t, tag; b, baseplate material). B, Thicken only over tags, leaving one thickness of wax elsewhere.

The lower baseplate presents special problems. Because of the shallowness of the lingual sulcus it is necessary to make lower plates sufficiently shallow also, and thus some extra thickness is often needed for strength.

In the molar region there is a deep lingual undercut extending to the root of the tongue. It is important not to carry tags into this undercut or to make the plate too thin in this region. It is generally necessary to ease lower plates in order to get them in and, if the plate is thin and is cut away from below or from the alveolar side, the tags are injured and the plate is unduly narrowed in a vertical direction.

If the plate is made thick enough beneath the tongue and the tags are brought vertically, it is then possible to ease the plate sufficiently to get it in by trimming it away laterally without reducing the depth of the plate or injuring the anchorage of the tags. There is also enough material to allow of finishing the bottom edge of the plate with a smooth round edge.

Another method is to block out the undercut first with plaster before making the plate (*Fig.* 21).

On the other hand, some practitioners make a lower plate as a small shallow rim of baseplate material. This gets over the difficulty of the lingual undercut in the molar region, but it results in a reduction in the space available for the disposition of tags.

Both in lower and in upper plates the importance cannot be too strongly emphasized of carefully rounding and polishing the free edge of the plate. This point is important, for it is a major factor in the comfort of the plate to the wearer.

THE PATIENT AND THE APPLIANCE

The success of orthodontic treatment depends so much on the co-operation of the patient that some consideration should be given to the patient's point of view and general attitude to treatment.

The frankly uncooperative patient is not so much an orthodontic problem as a psychological problem, and it is probably better to dismiss such patients with the understanding that if they subsequently undergo a change of heart their problem will be considered on its merits at that time without prejudice. Apart from this problem there is no reason why orthodontic treatment with removable appliances should not be completely successful within the limitations imposed by such appliances.

Patients are on the whole very tolerant of orthodontic appliances, however large and complicated they may be, and are prepared to put up with a good deal of inconvenience as a necessary part of their treatment. At the same time no pains should be spared to make all removable appliances comfortable, neat and unobtrusive. Baseplates should be as thin as possible consistent with adequate strength, bite planes should be no wider than is necessary to perform their proper functions. Neglect of these two points leads to the construction of appliances that encroach on the space required for the tongue, so disturbing the function of mastication and, more important to some patients, of speech. Patients very rapidly accommodate themselves to the wearing of appliances and most disturbances of speech and eating consequent on the insertion of appliances are soon overcome. The free edges of all baseplates, that is to say the lower and

so as to present a smooth aspect to any soft tissue that may lie against it (*Fig.* 120).

It is important not to make an appliance too complicated to insert, as an otherwise keen patient may be discouraged by repeated

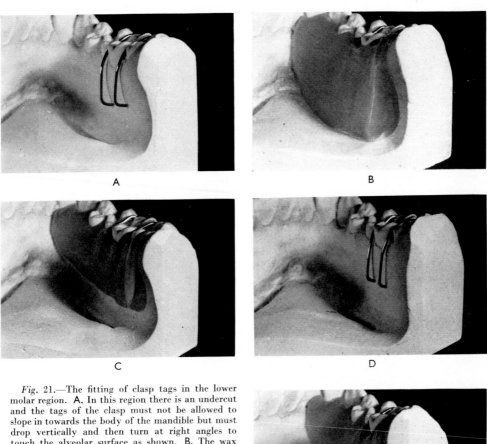

A

B

C

D

E

Fig. 21.—The fitting of clasp tags in the lower molar region. A, In this region there is an undercut and the tags of the clasp must not be allowed to slope in towards the body of the mandible but must drop vertically and then turn at right angles to touch the alveolar surface as shown. B, The wax baseplate must be trimmed vertically also, as shown, filling in the undercut area. C, When the baseplate is finished it is trimmed away from the mandibular side (shadow area) and the bottom edge of the plate rounded and smoothed. The appliance will then drop in without hurting the lingual gum margin of the lower teeth. D, As an alternative, the undercut area can be blocked in with plaster and the tags fitted vertically with normal length "turn ins" against the alveolar surface. E, The baseplate can then be made of correct thickness from the beginning.

posterior edges of lower baseplates and the posterior edges of upper baseplates, should be carefully rounded and polished. No spring should be left with sharp ends to irritate the lips or cheeks, but should be turned into a loop

difficulty in placing the appliance in position. At the same time it is often surprising to find how awkward an apparently bright patient is in putting in a quite simple appliance. It is necessary to have patience and to take

23

enough time to ensure that the patient understands exactly how to place and remove the appliance before sending him away. It is more satisfactory to leave the appliance entirely to the patient and never to invoke the assistance of a parent in placing and removing it. The patient will feel a sense of responsibility for the appliance and will be in a position to deal with it under all circumstances, and the time taken to educate him in the use of the appliance will thus be repaid over and over again. The patient who is dependent on a parent for inserting and removing his plate will never feel he is helping with treatment and will be at a loss if the appliance should come out or have to be removed when, for instance, he is at school or otherwise separated from the parent.

Appliances should be an *accurate fit*. This may seem a superfluous remark, but it is none the less necessary. If an appliance does not fit precisely when first put in it is most unlikely that it will come to fit with the passage of time, and if it does not fit it is also unlikely that it will work as it was designed to do. Appliances should be finished and placed in position within ten to fourteen days. The occlusion may be changing rapidly at the time at which orthodontic treatment is being carried out, and if there is much delay between taking the impression and fitting the appliance tooth movements can take place that may spoil the proper fitting of the appliance. This is particularly true where extractions have been recently carried out. In such circumstances drifting of teeth can be rapid and disastrous to the fitting of appliances. Where treatment involves extraction, it is almost always possible to make and fit removable appliances and allow the patient to get used to them for a day or so, before the extractions are performed.

Instructions to the patient should include most definite admonitions on the subject of oral hygiene while appliances are being worn. The ideal to be aimed at is thorough cleaning of the teeth, mouth, and appliance in the morning, last thing at night, and after every meal. This includes gentle brushing of the soft tissues of the gums and palate that are covered by the baseplates in order to make up for the loss of natural friction due to mastication and speech and so to keep these tissues fresh and healthy. Some patients appear to have no difficulty in keeping their mouths and appliances immaculately clean; others never appear to clean their teeth at all. If it is found that a patient is persistently neglectful of oral hygiene and shows an unusual tendency to periodontal disease or caries, the question should be carefully considered whether it is advisable to initiate or continue orthodontic treatment with appliances at all.

It is sometimes argued that some types of appliance are more or less hygienic than others, tending, as they may do, to collect less or more food debris as the case may be. It would seem, however, that it is not the gross food debris that becomes attached to wires that is likely to produce ill effects but the microscopic film of foodstuff that stagnates between the fitting surface of the appliance and the teeth and soft tissues, if the mouth and appliance are not cleaned after meals.

In order to reduce the area of sites of food stagnation about the teeth, it is sometimes advisable to thin down the edge of the baseplate, where it touches the teeth, to a very fine edge (*Fig.* 22). While this procedure is certainly necessary in some cases, it also has the attendant disadvantages that the edges of the plate are weakened and liable to break off, resulting in loss of fit and consequent loss of anchorage properties. The trimming of a baseplate in this way is difficult to perform without unintentionally easing the plate away from the teeth altogether with resulting loss of fit and hence of anchorage. An appliance also loses much of its support from the teeth unless it lies well and truly against their lingual surfaces. There is in fact no adequate substitute for adequate cleaning of the mouth and appliances at the appropriate times.

It is sometimes suggested that removable appliances need be worn at night time only. It is true that the Andresen appliance can only be worn at times when the patient is not engaged in normal day-time activities and the appliance is, therefore, of necessity limited to night-time use. The same arguments do

24

not, however, apply to removable appliances using springs or elastic traction. Such appliances do not interfere with normal ment to occur. In particular, there may be a tendency for spaces created in the buccal segments by extraction to close up from behind.

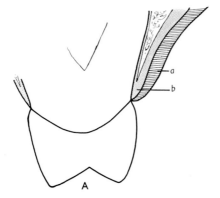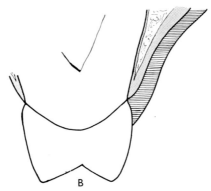

Fig. 22.—The fitting of baseplates to the lingual aspect of the teeth. **A**, This fitting is more hygienic as there is no stagnation area between the baseplate and the tooth. **B**, This fitting gives more positive support to the baseplate but it is necessary that the appliance and the mouth be kept clean. a, Baseplate. b, Palatal mucosa.

daytime activities if properly made, and most patients adapt themselves to wearing appliances quite rapidly. It is the author's experience that when appliances are worn for only one-third of the available time, i.e., at night only, tooth movement slows up to a very marked degree. Progress made during the night has a great tendency to relapse during the daytime. In many cases in which extractions have been performed there is a marked tendency for spontaneous tooth move-

Unless such spontaneous movement is carefully controlled by continuous wearing of an appliance the whole plan of treatment may be frustrated by undesired tooth movements. It is the author's practice, therefore, to make it a rule that appliances should be worn at all times, night, day, and at mealtimes, until treatment is complete. The only exception to this rule is that intermaxillary elastics must be removed at mealtimes, the appliances remaining in position.

CHAPTER III

THE MATERIALS FOR REMOVABLE APPLIANCE CONSTRUCTION

STAINLESS STEEL

STEEL wires have always been of great value for the construction of dental or orthodontic appliances, although the problems of rust and corrosion have placed limitations on their usefulness under the conditions met with in the mouth. In early dental literature piano wire was recommended where strength and elasticity were required, and the problem of corrosion was to some extent overcome by tinning the wire before use (Packham, 1932). The discovery of stainless steel and its eventual production in wire and ribbon form in Germany and Great Britain (Cutler, 1932) was followed by the development and refinement of methods for working, jointing, and exploiting the physical properties of the new material for orthodontic appliance construction (Friel, 1933).

Stainless steel is the material that is most widely used for the metallic parts of orthodontic appliance construction at the present time. The particular variety employed is known as 18/8 stainless steel alloy, containing 18 per cent chromium and 8 per cent nickel as major constituents.

Properties of Stainless Steel Wire.—The wires of the larger gauges, 0·6 mm. and upwards, are of a medium hardness which combines a useful elasticity for spring purposes with a degree of malleability that makes it possible to bend the wire with any desired degree of sharpness. It is important to remember that stainless steel wire must be worked and used in the state in which it is purchased. It is not feasible to alter the properties of the metal by heat treatment.★

A second important point is that stainless steel wire of medium hardness may be bent sharply and, if the bend is incorrectly placed, straightened out; but it may not be bent again at the same spot otherwise it will break, if not at the time, then before very long under conditions of use in the mouth. In other words, the material soon fatigues if *sharp* bends are overworked. The wire is, however, enormously strong if the mistake of overworking it is avoided. This means that when bending stainless steel wire a technique should be used which ensures the maximum accuracy in placing the bends and which will permit of adjustment of bends, after they have been made, without overworking the wire.

Soft stainless steel wires are available for use where spring and elasticity are not required or are actually undesirable. For instance, 0·7-mm. soft wire can be used for intermaxillary traction hooks. Although this wire is very soft and can be bent with spring-forming pliers, it is heavy enough to resist the pull of intermaxillary elastics (*Figs.* 145, 147). Fine soft wire, 0·3 mm. thick, may be used to bind together heavier wires before soldering or for ligatures in fixed appliance work.

Gauges of Wire.—Stainless steel wires of circular section are used in gauges of 1·0 mm. down to 0·15 mm. for the greater part of the wirework of most orthodontic appliances. Heavier gauges, 1·25 mm. and 1·5 mm., are used in a few situations. The thicker wires, 1·5 mm., 1·25 mm., 1·0 mm., 0·9 mm., and 0·8 mm., are used for bows and arches. The middle range, 0·7 mm. and 0·6 mm., are used for clasps and self-supporting springs. The

---

★ A new alloy known as "Elgiloy" has recently been developed in America. This alloy has been produced in wire form for orthodontic appliance construction. The

---

wire can be worked in the soft condition and then hardened by heat treatment.

thinner wires, 0·5 mm., 0·4 mm., 0·35 mm., and 0·3 mm., are used for finger springs and springs wound on supports or heavy arches. The very fine wires, 0·25 mm., 0·2 mm., and 0·15 mm., are used for coil springs, usually working on a heavier arch or support of some kind.

Orthodontists have become familiar with the use of stainless steel alloys for appliance construction, accepting the material as supplied by the manufacturer without specifying the manner of preparation, composition, or precise physical properties of the finished product, although Cutler (1932) described simple tests for evaluating the elasticity of wires and their resistance to breakage.

Stainless steel wires for orthodontic use are produced in three grades: very soft or fully

Table II.—CONVERSION TABLE FOR TENSILE STRENGTH*

DESCRIPTION	TENSILE STRENGTH		
	Lb./sq. in. (U.S.A.)	Tons/sq. in.	Kg./sq. mm.
Hard or Hard Drawn	224,000–246,400	100–110	157–173
	246,400–268,800	110–120	173–189
	268,800–291,200	120–130	189–205
	291,200–313,600	130–140	205–220
	313,600–336,000	140–150	220–236
High Tensile, Spring Hard, Super Hard	358,400 or more	160 or more	252 or more

annealed, hard, and a specially hard grade. The extra-hard grade may be called "high tensile", "spring hard", "super hard", or some similar term to indicate a specially hard wire.

For the usual hard grades of orthodontic stainless steel wire tensile strength varies from 100 to 150 tons per sq. in. depending on the thickness of the wire, the higher values relating to the finer grades of wire. The wires originally produced in Britain and used for orthodontic appliance construction were designated "hard" or "hard drawn". To-day, with the availability of wires from a number of manufacturers and the introduction of specially hard wires for fixed appliance arches, it is necessary to specify as accurately as possible the properties of the wires that should be used in removable

orthodontic construction. The use of an incorrect grade of wire may render the construction of appliances unnecessarily difficult if the wires are too hard, or prevent an appliance from working properly if the wires are too soft.

Table III.—TENSILE STRENGTH OF STAINLESS STEEL WIRES FOR ORTHODONTIC APPLIANCE CONSTRUCTION*

DIAMETER IN mm.	TENSILE STRENGTH IN tons/sq. in.	APPLICATION
1·5 1·25	100–110	Bows and arches
1·0 0·9 0·8	110–120	
0·7 0·6 0·5	120–130	}Clasps }Finger springs }Self-supporting springs
0·4 0·35 0·3	130–140	Springs supported on heavy arches
0·25 0·2 0·15	140–150	Twin-wire arch }Coil springs
0·4 0·45 0·5 0·55	160 or more	Arches for multiband appliances

* Extracts from British Standard 3507: (1962), "Specification for Orthodontic Wire and Tape and Dental Ligature Wire made of Stainless Steel" are reproduced by permission of the British Standards Institution, 2, Park Street, London, W.1, from whom copies of the complete standard may be purchased.

The British Specification 3507: 1962 specifies the properties of stainless steel wires and tapes for orthodontic use in regard to composition, size, tensile strength, resistance to failure on bending, and finish. If the properties of wires intended for orthodontic use are known in terms of the British Specification, no difficulty should be experienced in procuring suitable materials for any given purpose.

Tensile strength and resistance to failure on bending are the most practical means of defining the working properties of orthodontic wires. Tensile strength may be stated in kg. per sq. mm., lb. per sq. in. (U.S.A.), or tons per sq. in. The statement of tensile strength in tons per sq. in. gives a set of figures which is neat, concise, and easy to remember (*Table II*).

Wires having the tensile strengths shown in *Table III* provide the most suitable properties for the construction of removable orthodontic appliances.

HEAT TREATMENT OF STAINLESS STEEL WIRES

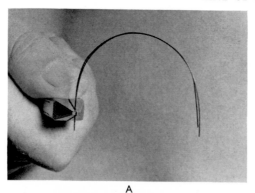

A

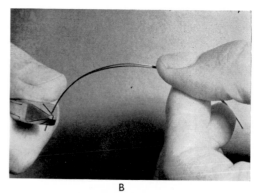

B

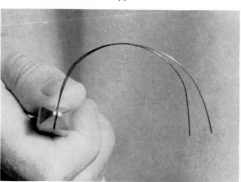

C

Fig. 23.—**A**, Two plain arches of 0·5-mm. hard wire have been formed. One has been heat-treated, the other has not. **B**, The archwires are held side by side in strong pliers and stroked once or twice with a straightening movement of the fingers and thumb. **C**, The heat-treated wire has resisted the straightening effect to a marked degree; the untreated wire has shown a tendency to return to its original shape before it was bent into arch form.

The possibility of heat-treating stainless steel for orthodontic applications has been known since 1949 (Backofen and Gales, 1952). These authors and Funk (1951) have shown experimentally that 18/8 hard drawn stainless steel wires may be successfully heat-treated after they have been formed into arches or loops. Heat treatment of wires before forming to the required shape does not enhance the physical properties. The effect of heat treating is shown in a simple way in *Fig.* 23 (Lager, 1963).

The Effects of Heat Treatment.—Heat treatment does not enhance the physical properties of stainless steel wires to any appreciable extent, as these properties are mainly derived by work-hardening during the wire drawing or metal rolling processes.

When such work-hardened wires are formed into arches or loops, however, further stresses occur at the points of bending, and it is these additional stresses that it is the purpose of heat treatment to remove. If this can be done without affecting the original physical properties of the material, arches and loops accept the new shape into which they have been bent, and resist deformation back towards their previous shape to a greater degree than they would if untreated. Such heat treatment is often referred to as "stress-relief anneal".

Applications of Stress-relieving Heat Treatment.—The value of heat treatment for arch wires used in multiband orthodontic appliances will be obvious, and such treatment applied to wires of similar gauges used as finger springs and auxiliary springs for removable appliances will confer corresponding benefits. The relief of stress in any wire which has been bent, especially if the bend is sharp and exposed to forces which may later lead to fracture, would be of value in clinical practice.

In the construction of removable appliances, the hard stainless steel wires may be used without any after-treatment. This is not to say that if simple and effective methods of heat treatment were at hand, improvements in removable appliance construction could not be made.

The Heat Treatment Procedures for Orthodontic Wires.—The obvious method for heat-treating wires is to place them in a temperature-controlled oven for a specified time. Backofen and Gales (1952) investigated the effect on stainless steel wires of heat treatment at 500°F. for 20 minutes and at 750°F. for 10 minutes, showing that the latter combination provides the better effect. These results do suggest, however, that a limitation on the use of the procedure is that it may not be convenient to heat-treat wires in an oven during the actual construction of an appliance because of the time involved.

An archwire may, however, be heat-treated almost instantly by passing an electric current through it. Provision for doing this is made on some orthodontic welders by means of two terminal blocks at which a potential of up to approximately 3–4 volts is available. The voltage is controlled by means of transformer tappings and a multipoint switch. One of the archwires shown in *Fig.* 23 was treated by applying 2·5 volts at the ends and carefully watching the colour of the wire. Within a matter of a few seconds the colour changed to a "medium straw", at which moment the current was switched off and heat treatment was complete. For finer wires or arches having loops or coils, being therefore longer, a higher potential than 2·5 volts would be required to overcome the electrical resistance and to cause the passage of a current adequate to generate the necessary heat.

The heat treatment of springs and clasps for removable appliance construction could be made a practical proposition by preforming these parts and "soaking" them in a gas or electric oven for 10 minutes at 750° F. The effectiveness of the procedure in terms of improved resilience of the wires would need to be assessed largely in the light of clinical experience.

MILLIMETRES OR INCHES

The dimensions of orthodontic materials can be stated in thousandths of an inch or in millimetres. The standard wire gauge is rarely if ever used to-day in orthodontics.

Table IV.—WIRE AND TAPE THICKNESS IN MILLIMETRES AND EQUIVALENT THICKNESS IN INCHES

mm.	inches	inches	thous of an inch
1·5	0·05906	0·059	60
1·25	0·04921	0·049	50
1·0	0·03937	0·039	40
0·9	0·03543	0·035	36
0·8	0·03150	0·032	32
0·7	0·02756	0·028	28
0·65	0·02559	0·026	26
0·6	0·02362	0·024	24
0·55	0·02165	0·022	22
0·5	0·01968	0·020	20
0·45	0·01772	0·018	18
0·4	0·01575	0·016	16
0·35	0·01378	0·014	14
0·3	0·01181	0·012	12
0·25	0·00984	0·010	10
0·2	0·00787	0·008	8
0·15	0·00591	0·006	6
0·1	0·00394	0·004	4
0·05	0·00197	0·002	2
0·025	0·00098	0·001	1

The choice of the British or the metric scale depends as a rule on custom or upbringing, but it is useful to understand the relationship between the two scales so that either may be used at will and measurements transposed from one scale to the other when required.

One metre is equal to 39·37 inches, from which it follows that 1·0 mm. = 0·03937 in. In *Table IV* the first column gives the sizes of wires commonly used, in millimetres; the second column shows the equivalent size in inches to five decimal places; the third shows the sizes in inches correct to three decimal places.

If the approximation is accepted that for practical purposes 1·0 mm. = 0·04 in. the conversion of millimetres to inches becomes even simpler and the calculations can be made mentally.

In the fourth column sizes of the wires are given as worked out from the approximation that 1·0 mm. = 40 thousandths of an inch. The differences between these figures and the values correct to three decimal places are very slight and only occur in the heaviest gauges of wire.

Finally, it is useful to keep in mind when thinking of thicknesses of wire that for practical purposes:—

1 millimetre = 40 thousandths of an inch.

1 thousandth of an inch = 0·025 millimetre.

THE ACRYLIC RESINS

The acrylic resins, both heat-curing and self-curing, are used for the construction of baseplates and of the screens of functional appliances.

Heat-curing Acrylic Resins.—Heat-curing resins give as a final product a dense, hard, colour-stable plate free from porosity and, if colourless polymer is used, a clear transparent material. The appliance must be preformed in wax and invested and the resin processed in the flask under heat and pressure.

A great deal of time and effort can be saved if the wax-up stage of the appliance and the process of investment are carefully done by following a few straightforward methods.

1. The wire parts of the appliance should be fixed to the dry dental cast with a minimum of pink wax, filling the spaces between the tags and the plaster. (*Fig.* 24 A.)

2. The dental cast is then briefly dipped in water and surface wetness is allowed to dry. Pink wax flowed on to the cast will then adhere but can be trimmed and the excess picked cleanly off giving an accurate outline to the waxed-up appliance.

3. Wax is then applied to the cast as a single sheet sufficiently softened and pressed down to the upper model without thinning out the palate. In the lower arch, extra thickness is applied where necessary. (*Fig.* 24 B, C.)

4. The wax is firmly pressed down around the teeth and trimmed to shape with a flat-ended plastic filling instrument. The wax is also trimmed around springs. (*Fig.* 24 D.)

5. The edges of the wax around the teeth and springs are quickly flamed, pressed into accurate contact with the plaster and given a final trim, if necessary using a No. 12 probe around the coils of any springs. (*Fig.* 24 E.)

6. When flasking the appliance care should be taken to put plaster accurately around the springs and inside the coils. If an air bubble forms inside a coil, the resin which goes into it subsequently is not easy to remove without damaging the wire.

7. When processed the appliance is deflasked and all plaster removed; it is only necessary to take away the flask using an acrylic bur and to polish the plate. If trimming to shape or thickness has to be done the appliance could not have been properly waxed up or invested or both. Dental burs should *never* be used to free spring coils or guides from the baseplate. If acrylic material has been allowed to encroach on such wires, it should be carefully pared back with a sharp vulcanite chisel and the coil finally freed by placing a probe through the coil and rocking it just enough to free the wire from the embrace of the resin to allow the coil to act.

Self-curing Acrylic Materials.—Even when the best methods of waxing, packing, and finishing are used, the construction of appliances in heat-curing acrylic resin takes time. The use of self-polymerizing acrylic materials makes it possible to repair and adjust orthodontic appliances without the need to follow the normal procedure of waxing-up, flasking, packing, and finishing in the laboratory. It is also possible, using this material, to construct complete appliances rapidly and conveniently (Hallett, 1952; Weber, 1960; Cousins, 1962).

Clasps, arches, or springs are constructed in the usual way, and placed in position on the working model which has been previously coated with a film of the appropriate separating material. The clasps are secured in position with a little pink wax, attached on the buccal side, leaving the palatal or lingual area over

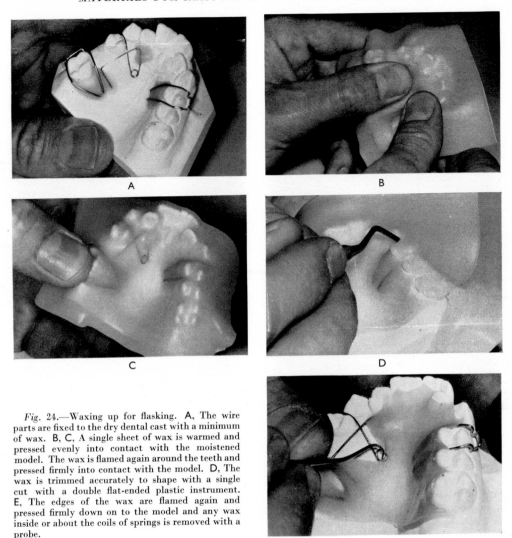

Fig. 24.—Waxing up for flasking. **A,** The wire parts are fixed to the dry dental cast with a minimum of wax. **B, C,** A single sheet of wax is warmed and pressed evenly into contact with the moistened model. The wax is flamed again around the teeth and pressed firmly into contact with the model. **D,** The wax is trimmed accurately to shape with a single cut with a double flat-ended plastic instrument. **E,** The edges of the wax are flamed again and pressed firmly down on to the model and any wax inside or about the coils of springs is removed with a probe.

which the baseplate must extend clear. Parts of springs which must not be bound up in the baseplate material are covered with pink wax, which will also help to hold them in place, and when the wax has set it is accurately trimmed to cover up only that part of the springs that must be left free in the finished appliance (*Fig.* 25).

The self-curing acrylic material is then applied to the model. This may be done either by running or pressing on a thin mixture of the material, or the powder and liquid may be added separately, building up the thickness of the baseplate as may be required (*Fig.* 26). In order to avoid the need for extensive carving of the baseplate after the acrylic material has hardened, care should be taken to see that excessive bulk does not accumulate in the vault of the palate in an upper model. This area is sometimes difficult to get at to trim and polish if the dental arch is narrow and the palatal vault relatively high. The movement of the soft material can be controlled by positioning the model and by constructing the baseplate in sections, thereby avoiding the difficulty of having material flowing from two directions into a central pool.

When the required area and thickness of the material have been applied to the working model, setting can be accelerated by placing the completed appliance in warm water. The polymerizing of the material can be accelerated

fit of appliances made in one material or in the other.

The disadvantages associated with the use of self-curing acrylics are that the material may suffer from the drawbacks of difficulty in obtaining a high polish, a tendency to porosity, and colour instability. These problems can be overcome to a great extent by processing the

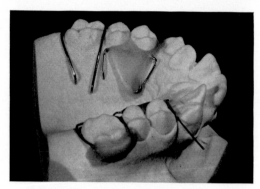

Fig. 25.—Clasps and springs are attached to the model with pink wax. For the springs, the pink wax serves to block out areas which do not need to be reproduced in acrylic material and also holds the wires in place.

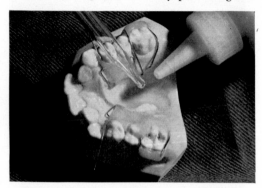

Fig. 26.—Liquid is dropped on with a dropper and the powder blown on from a soft polythene bottle. Note that the position of the model controls the flow of the acrylic mixture. One side of an appliance should be completed and have begun to set before the other is commenced. For the construction of the front part of the baseplate, the model is placed with the incisors downwards.

and porosity eliminated by applying warmth and pressure simultaneously in a hydraulic pressure flask. The appliance is removed from the model, trimmed to shape, and polished in the usual way, care being taken to avoid overheating on the lathe brush. It is sometimes claimed that appliances made in this way fit more accurately than appliances made with heat-curing acrylic, but it is very doubtful whether there is a significant difference in the

appliance by the hydraulic pressure flask technique. It is also sometimes found that the oral tissues are sensitive to these materials. Where speed is essential and large numbers of appliances are required regularly from a laboratory the use of self-curing acrylic materials may be a valuable contribution to the treatment of patients.

CHAPTER IV

ORTHODONTIC TECHNIQUE

ORTHODONTIC technique is essentially a matter of skill in the bending of wire. The importance to the orthodontist of gaining adequate skill and facility in the art of bending wire cannot be overstressed, but all too often the development of individual capacity in this direction is left entirely to chance. Occasionally an operator will acquire a high degree of skill

methods of bending wire are never discovered and applied. It may, therefore, be useful to discuss the nature of wire-bending problems and how they may best be overcome.

WIRE-BENDING METHOD

The problem of bending wires to the various shapes required for orthodontic purposes has

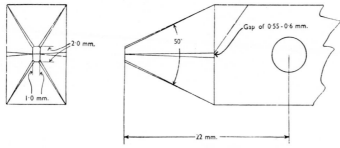

Fig. 27.—Universal pliers. The blades of these pliers must be accurately ground to the dimensions indicated. The tips of the beaks should not be less in size than shown, but may be slightly more if the metal is not adequately hard and tough.

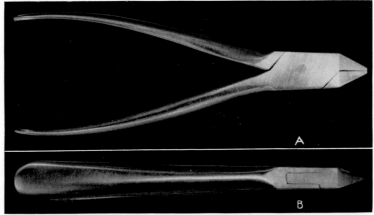

Fig. 28.—A, Universal pliers measure 5¼ in. overall and have gracefully curved handles designed for a maximum pressure with minimum expenditure of energy. B, The handles are comfortably broad to distribute the pressure over a wide area of the palm and fingers.

and work out a rationale of wire bending for himself over the course of years, but as a rule much time is wasted and the best and easiest

been tackled in the past in two ways. Over the course of many years a long succession of orthodontists have devised a multitude of special pliers each designed to serve some particular wire-bending purpose. Such pliers are made with specially formed beaks, grooves, serrations, or additional parts about which the wire can be bent, so making the bending operation simple and almost automatic. In some types of pliers simply grasping the wire firmly between the beaks will produce the required bend.

of wire bending either to multiply his stock of pliers to widen the range of bends he can make or else to limit his technical procedures to the limitations of his pliers. Special pliers are sometimes limited in the thickness of wire they can bend.

These physical limitations of specialized pliers may also impose a limitation on the imagination of their user through a failure on

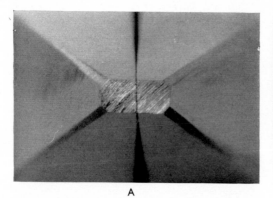 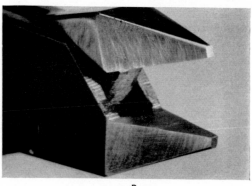

A   B

Fig. 29.—A, The tips of the pliers are ground very accurately to 1·5 mm. square. The outer corners are slightly chamfered. B, The inner surfaces of the beaks are not polished; the edges of the beaks are quite sharp and must not be bevelled or rounded.

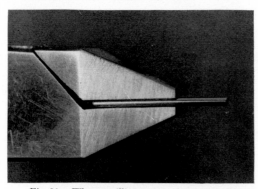

Fig. 30.—When a millimetre wire is grasped the inside surfaces of the beaks are parallel.

Specialized pliers certainly have the advantage that they will perform the bending operation for which they are designed quickly and easily, but they have corresponding and outweighing disadvantages. Most special pliers perform only one or two operations; the more specialized the pliers the fewer the bends that can be performed. Consequently there is a tendency for an operator who uses this method

his part to appreciate the possibilities of applied basic wire-bending method in the construction of appliances.

The alternative approach to wire-bending problems is based on three foundations. Firstly, the use of one or two basically simple pliers; secondly, the study of wire-bending methods; and, thirdly, the elimination of unnecessary complications from wire work in appliance construction.

Adams Universal Pliers.—Wire-bending is greatly simplified if the number of pliers used is reduced to the essential minimum. Universal pliers (*Fig.* 28), in conjunction with a study and application of wire-bending principles, will perform every wire-bending operation required for removable appliance construction, with the exception of the formation of loops in finger springs and other cantilever springs.

The essential features of these pliers are:—

1. The distance between the hinge pin and the tips of the blades is short: 22 mm. is the optimum length.

34

2. The handles are large, comfortable, and as long as possible consistent with comfort to the user's hand. In particular, it should be possible to place the thumb of the hand gripping the handles on or very near the tip of the blades, while at the same time applying a strong grip (*Figs.* 35, 45, 58).

3. The taper of the blades should be accurately ground to the angle shown.

4. The sides of the beaks should be perfectly flat.

5. The outer edges of the blades are very slightly chamfered, but not rounded (*Figs.* 27, 29).

of the beaks are parallel. It is thus possible to grasp a 1·0-mm. wire with the whole length of the beaks, so securing a powerful grip. Again, when a wire is grasped only at the tips of the beaks, the tendency for the wire to shoot out from the beaks is greatly reduced (*Fig.* 30).

9. The hinge of the pliers should be strong without being too bulky and the handles large and comfortable without making the pliers heavy and clumsy to handle. An overall length of $5\frac{1}{4}$ in. is about right.

These pliers depend for their action on the power with which it is possible to grasp the

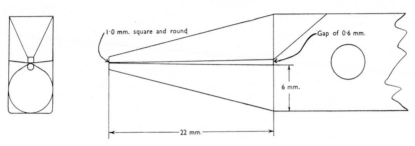

Fig. 31.—Spring-forming pliers. Should be accurately ground to dimensions shown. The tips should be at most 1·0 mm. square and round in size, but may be less if desired and if the quality of the metal will permit.

6. The edges of the grasping surfaces of the beaks must be left sharp after the final grinding operation in manufacture and *must not be bevelled at all*. This point is very important. (*Figs.* 29, 34.)

7. The grasping surfaces of the beaks should be matt finished. *They must not be polished* but equally they must not be grooved or serrated. The finish left by fine filing or grinding is satisfactory provided that the subsequent chromium plating is not polished either. Sometimes the grasping surfaces of the beaks will be found to have been coated with a fine metallic dust. This provides an exceedingly satisfactory surface (*Fig.* 29B).

8. When the pliers are closed, the tips of the beaks should be in contact, but there should be a slight gap at the hinge end of the beaks tapering down evenly to contact at the tips. This gap should be 0·55–0·6 mm. at its widest part, so that when the tips of the beaks are open to 1·0 mm. the inner surfaces

wire with a moderate hand pressure. A slight additional grip is given by the sharp edges of the beaks when the wire is bent. The absence of serrations on the beaks avoids injury to the wire, and the absence of grooves and nicks makes it possible to grasp the wire in an infinite number of positions. Grooving the beaks of pliers makes them into special pliers and greatly limits their usefulness.

Universal pliers will bend any of the wires used for orthodontic purposes with ease and are particularly useful for clasp construction (*see* Chapter V).

Correction and Maintenance of Adams Universal Pliers.—The specification of these pliers is simple and if the pliers are correctly made in the first instance the accurate bending of wire and the construction of clasps will be found to be quick and easy to perform. All too often, however, Adams universal pliers are produced with lack of attention to some points in the specification and in consequence wires can only be held with difficulty and effort, and the user quickly becomes fatigued and irritated with his lack of technical success.

Faults that may be met with in these pliers are that they may be made of stainless steel, they may be too long or too short in overall

ground back carefully by holding them against a fine grinding wheel on a dental lathe run at low speed (*Fig.* 29A).

If the inner surfaces of the beaks have been polished in manufacture the polish must be removed using a very small mounted stone in a

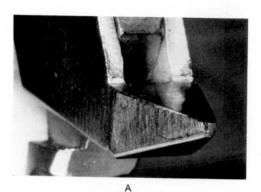

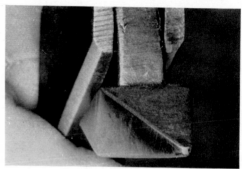

A   B

Fig. 32.—Faults in production. A, There is a polish in the grasping surfaces of the beaks and the grasping edges are bevelled. B, The grasping surfaces of these pliers are correctly matt finished but there is a very large bevel on the grasping edges. Both these pliers are new and unused. The first set is virtually useless and the second pliers require correction before use.

length, or the beaks may be polished on the grasping surfaces and the inner edges of the beaks may be bevelled or rounded. (*Fig.* 32.)

The form of the beaks may easily be corrected by carefully grinding off the sides just sufficiently to make a sharp edge. To do this with a grinding wheel on a motor is a difficult operation for the uninitiated because there is no room for the slightest mistake. The sides of the beaks must be left flat and the slope towards the tips must not be altered. It is clear that material must be ground off uniformly over the whole surface.

While the correction can be made on a grinding machine, it is altogether more satisfactory to do the job using a small jig (*Fig.* 33 A, B) and rubbing down the beaks on a fine carborundum stone under a stream of water to keep the stone clean and cutting freely. In this way the operation can be done with complete certainty in a matter of minutes. By the same method the top and bottom surfaces and the bevel on the outer corners can be touched up (*Fig.* 33 C, D, E).

If, after these adjustments, the tips of the beaks are found to be too fine they should be

straight handpiece. It is, of course, vital that the grasping surfaces of the beaks should be flat and great care should be taken not to round these surfaces in the slightest degree.

The adjustments that have been mentioned may, of course, be carried out on pliers that have been in use for a period of years and have become worn at the edges and smooth on the grasping surfaces of the jaws (*Fig.* 34). Stainless steel wire is a very tough material to fabricate and plier beaks inevitably show signs of wear in time. Well made and hardened steel pliers will last for years, but if the metal is not good or properly hardened wear will soon show up in use.

Spring-forming Pliers.—The only other essential pliers for removable-appliance construction are spring-forming pliers. There are many patterns available, but those illustrated in *Fig.* 31 have distinct advantages. For instance, anything from a tiny coil in a 0·3-mm. wire to a large coil in a 0·7-mm. wire can be formed. Again, coils can be opened and adjusted by placing the square beak as far into the coil as possible and gently closing the round beak on the outside of the coil.

36

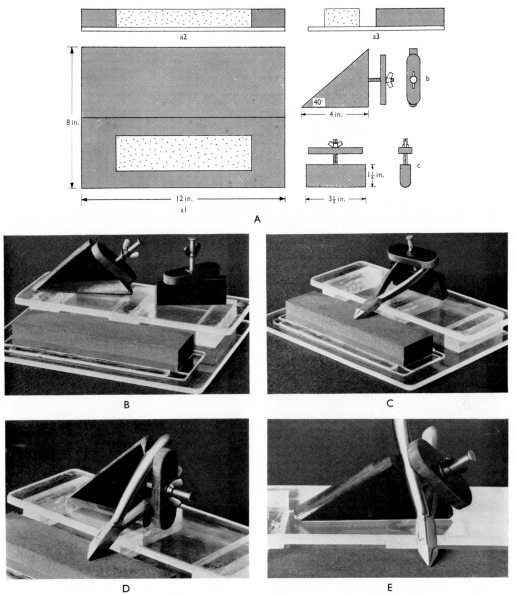

Fig. 33.—The correction and maintenance of Adams universal pliers. This can be done with a simple jig for grinding pliers at the correct angles. **A**, The essential dimensions of the plier trimming jig are given in this diagram. The carborundum stone should be of medium grade and measure $8 \times 2 \times 1$ in. The baseboard measures 12×8 in. and the raised platform is the same thickness as the stone. The views of the baseboard are: a1 plan, a2 front elevation, a3 end-view. The jigs for guiding the pliers are shown at **b** and **c**. The screws are $\frac{1}{4}$ in. Whitworth, brass, with a washer and wing nut. The entire jig can be made of wood if it is only used occasionally, but as it is necessary to use much water when grinding it is better to use Perspex or Tufnol which are not affected by damp. In the photographs it can be seen that the raised platform is not solid but is built up in three places by means of strips of material to the correct thickness. The carborundum stone is held in place by strips of Perspex cemented to the baseboard. **B**, A general view of the jig and grindstone. The pliers are clamped, using the wing nuts, at the correct angles for grinding as in **C, D, E. C**, Grinding the sides. The beaks are rubbed all over the surface of the stone to avoid hollowing of the surface with time. **D**, Grinding the top or bottom. **E**, Grinding the bevel.

It is important when using spring-forming pliers to relate thickness of the wire being bent to the point along the blade of the pliers that is being used to make the bend will depend on the strength and quality of the pliers. The use of spring-forming pliers to make sharp bends in heavy wires is one of the most common abuses of pliers.

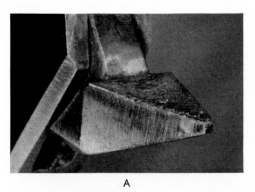
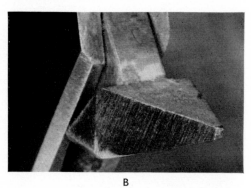

Fig. 34.—The correction of pliers that are bevelled or worn at the grasping edges. A, Adams universal pliers after some years of use; note the turning over of the working edges. B, The same pliers after grinding the sides of the beaks. Note the straight sharp edge of the beak.

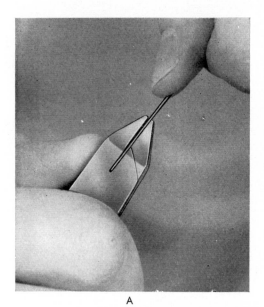
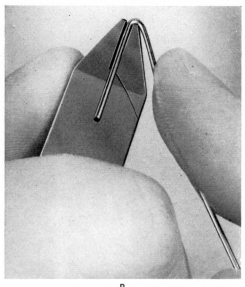

Fig. 35.—Making a sharp bend in heavy wire using Adams universal pliers. The wire is held so that it is grasped by the whole length of the plier beaks and the bend is made over the corner of the tip of one beak using the thumb to exert firm pressure. (This operation is seen from the spectator's point of view, i.e., the left hand is on the right of the picture.)

and not to bend too thick a wire too near to the tips of the pliers. It is not possible to lay down any other rule on this matter, as much

One of the most important features of pliers is that they should be made of good steel, well hardened. Properly made pliers will last indefinitely without wearing. Inferior pliers wear rapidly, require frequent trimming and adjusting, and eventually wear out.

Heavy stainless steel wires are difficult to bend because the material is strong and tough and because it is necessary to bend the wire sharply and with great accuracy. The

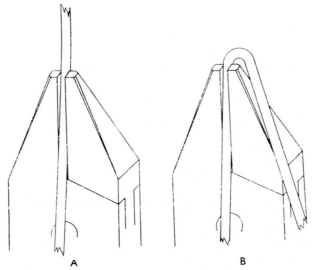

Fig. 36.—Diagrammatic representation of *Fig.* 35 showing relation of wire and pliers.

Problems in the Bending of Wire and Their Solution.—The bending of fine wires does not present much difficulty as the resistance of these wires to bending is slight in comparison with the strength of the fingers and the finest of fine spring-forming pliers.

basic difficulties in bending heavy stainless steel wires are therefore:—

1. The making of sharp bends in heavy wires.
2. The accurate placing of such bends.
3. The construction of complicated shapes for bows, arches, and clasps.

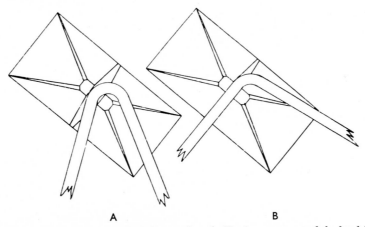

Fig. 37.—The correction of sharp bends in heavy wire. A, The incorrect part of the bend is grasped in the tips of Adams universal pliers and squeezed firmly. B, This will straighten this portion of the wire. The sharp edges of the beaks of the pliers prevent the wire from slipping but do not injure the wire. The wire is then bent where required.

39

The principles and methods of wire-forming are few and simple and are as follows:—

1. An adequate length of wire should be used so that a long end or "tail" is available for manipulation, while the formed part of the wire is held in the pliers and so away from any possibility of accidental distortion.

2. The pliers should be used to hold the wire firmly and still. The wire is then bent, using the long free end or "tail" for this and squeezed. This has the effect of straightening the small section of wire selected without interfering with the remainder of the bend, which may, in fact, be just as it was intended to be. The wire is then re-bent at the correct spot at the other side of the remainder of the original bend. This method of correcting bends is better than straightening the whole bend and starting again as this is liable to overstress the wire and render it crystalline

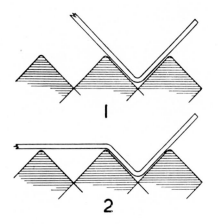
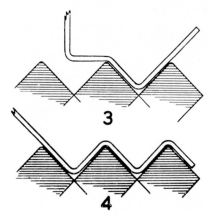

Fig. 38.—Bending wire into corners. Exercises 2 and 3. The secret is to pre-form the bend that is to be worked into the corner. The left-hand bend (Stage 3) is formed and then turned down to fit into the corner (Stage 4). If it is not certain where to make this bend (Stage 3) make it a little short of the corner in Stage 4 and then, by applying a correction as in *Fig.* 37, the bend can be worked down accurately into the corner.

purpose. Bends can be made much more accurately and sharply than if the wire is held still and bent by moving the pliers.

3. It should always be arranged that the free end of the wire is held in the hand in such a way that the thumb is used to bring pressure on the wire, the other fingers being wrapped around and grasping the wire. The wire should be bent with the *thumb*; the fingers are not so strong and cannot apply such a strong and controlled pressure.

4. Sharp bends are made by bending the wire over the corner of the end of the plier blade, *not round the end of the blade* (*Figs.* 35 A, B, 36 A, B).

5. If the wire has been sharply bent at a slightly incorrect position, a correction may be made if the wire is straightened as indicated in *Fig.* 37 A, B. The incorrect portion of the bend is gripped in the tips of the plier beaks

and very liable to break under the forces it later encounters in the mouth.

6. The bending of 0·7-mm. wire sharply as required for the modified arrowhead clasp should be carefully studied (*see* pp. 52–57). These bends are not made around the ends of the plier beaks at all but are made *outside* the tips of the beaks.

7. Smooth bends are made from a large number of small bends.

8. The working of a wire into corners requires a method that is illustrated in *Fig.* 38. This kind of bend is often required when constructing lingual arches and it is required to fit some part into interdental spaces. The principle in brief is to prefabricate the bend that fits in the corner and gradually work it down into place.

9. When constructing bows or arches to fit *outside* a model, make the arch too wide and

gradually contract it to fit. When constructing bows or arches to fit *inside* a model, make the arch too narrow and gradually expand it to fit. In both cases the principle is the same.

The wire must be made *too loose* and gradually worked down to a fit. If the wire is too tight it is never possible to see exactly where it is binding and where to make the necessary correction.

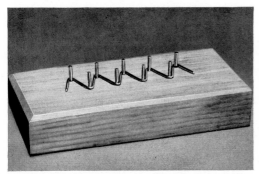

Fig. 39.—Exercise No. 1. The pins are thick gramophone needles set ½ in. apart; the rows of pins are also ½ in. apart.

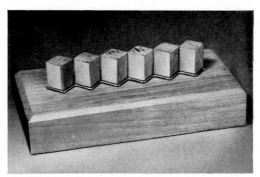

Fig. 40.—Exercise No. 2. The posts are square and ½ in. diagonal. The corners against which the wire is fitted are *very slightly* rounded, it being impossible to make a perfectly sharp angle in 1·0-mm. wire.

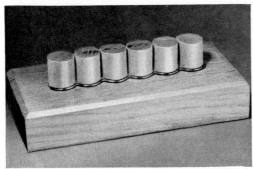

Fig. 41.—Exercise No. 3. The posts are ½ in. in diameter and ½ in. high.

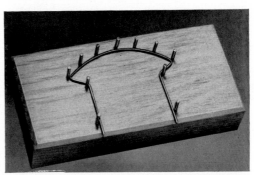

Fig. 42.—Exercise No. 4. Simple lingual arch prototype.

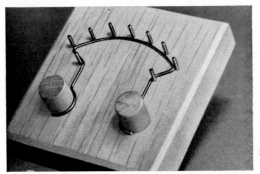

Fig. 43.—Exercise No. 5. Lingual arch prototype. The posts are ½ in. in diameter.

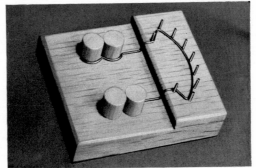

Fig. 44.—Exercise No. 6. Difficult lingual arch prototype. The step in the block makes the arch three dimensional. The step is ¼ in. deep. The posts are ½ in. in diameter.

Wire bending is conveniently taught and practised on a special set of geometrical models which are specially designed to illustrate basic principles (*Figs.* 39–44). These models are made of small hardwood blocks into some of which steel pins are driven, others having square or round posts. Others again have pins and posts fixed into them. The placing and arrangement of these pins and posts is done according to a definite plan and pattern and not just in a haphazard way.

The first exercise consists of bending wire so as to fit exactly around two rows of pins in a zig-zag manner. This requires accurate placing of sharp turns in the wire and the method of adjusting the position of a sharp turn in a heavy wire as already explained is essential to the successful performance of this exercise.

The second exercise, consisting of six square pegs, makes use of the principle of working wire into corners or angles between objects as already shown. The third exercise is made with round pegs instead of square pegs, and is hence a little more difficult than the second, but the principle is the same.

The last three exercises are lingual arch prototypes of increasing degrees of difficulty. They exhibit nothing further in wire-bending principle apart from the art of securing passivity in a lingual arch or bow.

All these exercises are performed with 1·0-mm. stainless steel wire using Adams universal pliers only, and when completed should conform to the following requirements:—

1. The wires must fit around exactly or touch all pins and fit closely around all posts.

2. The wires must lie perfectly flat on the wood blocks.

3. The wire must be perfectly passive and should fall off the block when it is inverted and gently shaken (Nos. 1, 4, 5, 6).

4. The wires should not be so loose that they rattle when the blocks are shaken (Nos. 1, 4, 5, 6).

When carrying out these exercises an important point is to check the fit of the wire *after every bend* and to correct mistakes as they arise. Inaccuracies must not be allowed to accumulate; this is a most important principle, as it is futile to try to correct a discrepancy due to a recent bend by going back beyond this point and interfering with the early part of the exercise which is correct.

A series of exercises of this kind is useful not only for the student who has to learn the fundamentals of wire-bending method from the beginning, but also for the enthusiast who wishes to check his methods and skill and strengthen and speed up his technique. The exercises are not devised primarily in order to test and tease the performer but to illustrate principles in wire-forming and to give the opportunity for their practice. The exercise blocks are automatically critical of every performance because, being geometrical and accurate, there can be no two opinions as to whether an exercise has been accurately performed or not. The most casual glance and inversion of the block will tell all that has to be known. The performer, therefore, has a constant and accurate standard to aim at and one that can in fact be achieved with a little patience and practice.

APPLIED WIRE-BENDING TECHNIQUE

Adams universal pliers will be found useful in a great variety of situations such as, for instance, the bending of heavy wires for all purposes, for clasp construction, and for holding wires while being worked on by some other pliers or instrument. (*Figs.* 45, 47.)

Adams spring-forming pliers are satisfactory for the formation of loops in wire of varying thicknesses up to 1·0 mm. Care should be taken when bending the heavier wires to use the strongest part of the beaks near to the hinge of the pliers. It would be unreasonable, for instance, to expect to bend a hard 1·0-mm. wire using the tips of the beaks. The finer wires, 0·4 mm. and smaller, can be bent at any point on the beaks.

Sometimes the entire bending and adaptation of the spring can be effected using the spring-forming pliers, but in many instances a firmer and easier grip may be obtained with the Adams universal pliers for formation, finishing, and adjusting of springs. (*Figs.* 48, 49.)

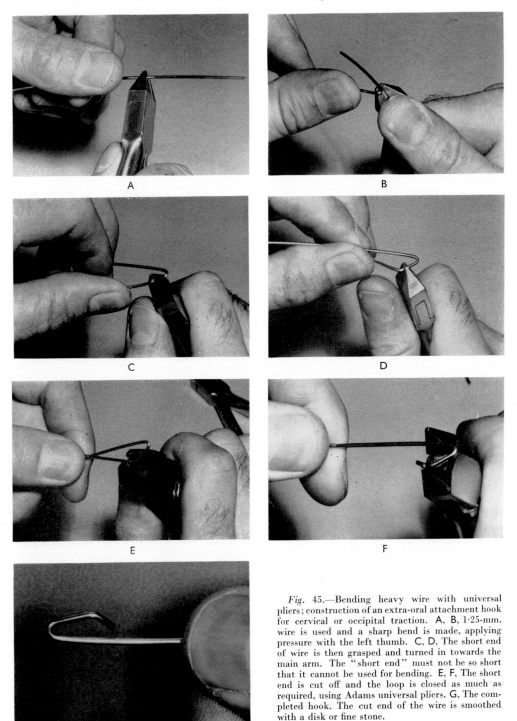

Fig. 45.—Bending heavy wire with universal pliers; construction of an extra-oral attachment hook for cervical or occipital traction. A, B, 1·25-mm. wire is used and a sharp bend is made, applying pressure with the left thumb. C, D, The short end of wire is then grasped and turned in towards the main arm. The "short end" must not be so short that it cannot be used for bending. E, F, The short end is cut off and the loop is closed as much as required, using Adams universal pliers. G, The completed hook. The cut end of the wire is smoothed with a disk or fine stone.

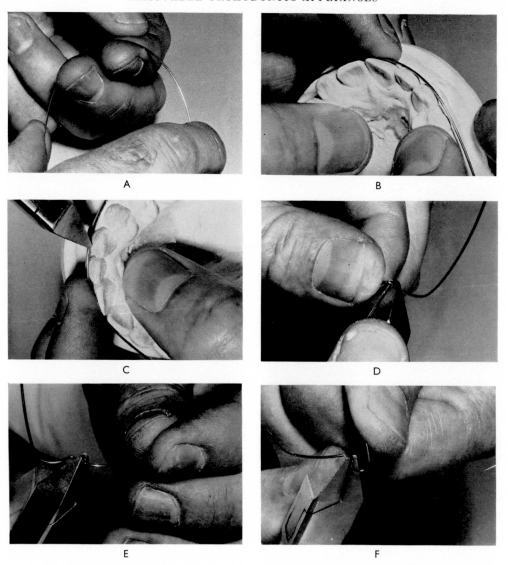

A

B

C

D

E

F

Fig. 47.

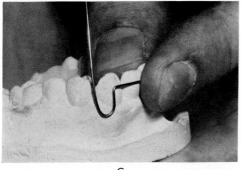

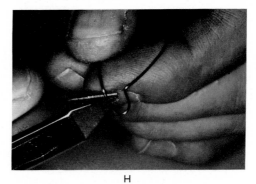

G

H

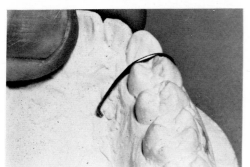

Fig. 46.—Bending medium wire with Adams universal pliers. Making a labial bow with U loops as for an Andresen appliance or a retainer. A, B, 7-mm. wire is used and the first smooth curve is made with the fingers and the wire adapted to the labial surface of the upper six anterior teeth. C, U loop is started by bending the wire up at right angles at the centre of the canine tooth; the point is marked by grasping the wire in the pliers. D, The 90° bend is made. E, The curve of the U loop is started, the labial bow is on the left. F, The U loop is finished using Adams universal pliers. G, The U loop is tried on the cast. H, The tag is brought over the embrasure towards the palate. I, The finishing of the tag in the palate.

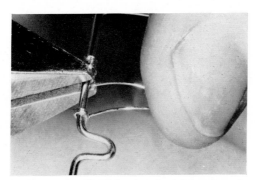

Fig. 47.—Bending light wire using Adams universal pliers; adjusting an apron spring. The coils of the spring are immobilized by grasping gently in the pliers while the position of the apron is adjusted by bending with the left index finger (on right).

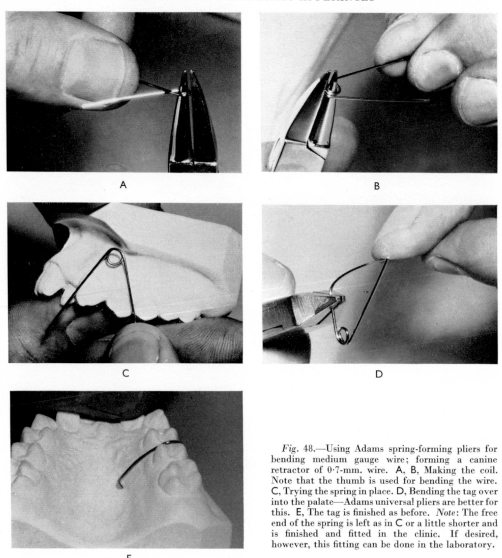

A

B

C

D

E

Fig. 48.—Using Adams spring-forming pliers for bending medium gauge wire; forming a canine retractor of 0·7-mm. wire. **A, B,** Making the coil. Note that the thumb is used for bending the wire. **C,** Trying the spring in place. **D,** Bending the tag over into the palate—Adams universal pliers are better for this. **E,** The tag is finished as before. *Note*: The free end of the spring is left as in **C** or a little shorter and is finished and fitted in the clinic. If desired, however, this fitting can be done in the laboratory.

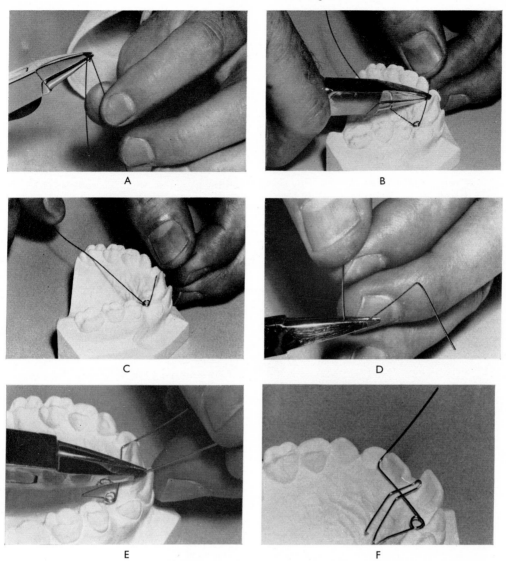

Fig. 49.—Manipulating fine wire with spring-forming pliers. Making a finger spring of 0·5-mm. wire to procline an upper incisor tooth. A, A single coil is placed in the wire. B, The spring is tried in place and the free end marked by grasping in the pliers. C, The free end is turned round the tooth to be moved. D, The tag end is turned down into the palate at the coil and brought back again across the spring to form the guide. E, The tag end is marked for length by grasping with the pliers and turned back into the palate, completing the tag. F, The completed spring.

CHAPTER V

THE DESIGN AND CONSTRUCTION OF ORTHODONTIC CLASPS

Clasps of any kind depend for their action on the existence of undercuts or retentive surfaces in the shape of the teeth. The clasp material is made to fit below such undercuts and grip the tooth so that displacement of the appliance bearing the clasps is resisted. The

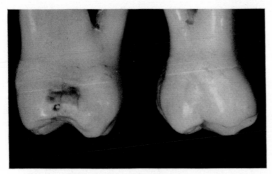

Fig. 50.—The right upper first permanent molar. On left, mesial aspect, on right, buccal aspect.

THE RETENTIVE SURFACES OF TEETH

The upper first permanent molar illustrates well the available retentive surfaces of a tooth (*Figs.* 50, 51). The buccal and lingual undercuts are apparent from the mesial aspect of the tooth. The buccal surface of the molar is, in the main, flat, but just at the cervical margin there is a small undercut amounting almost to a ridge of enamel in this situation. The lingual surface is more bulbous, and towards the anatomical neck of the tooth there is a distinct undercut. Both these undercuts are most marked at the anatomical neck of the tooth and are not visible or usable for appliance-retention purposes until the tooth is fully erupted (*Fig.* 51 A).

The mesial and distal undercuts are visible from the buccal aspect of the molar (*Fig.* 51 B). It will be noticed that the widest mesiodistal diameter of the tooth is at the level

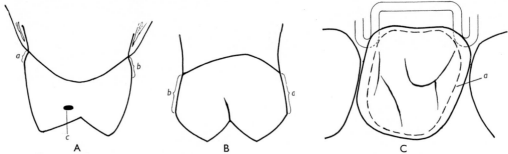

Fig. 51.—The retentive surfaces of upper right first permanent molar: A, Mesial aspect: a, Buccal undercut; b, Lingual undercut; c, Contact point. B, Buccal aspect: a, Mesial undercut; b, Distal undercut. C, Occlusal aspect: a, Anatomical neck. Note that the mesial and distal undercuts extend buccally and are accessible to the arrowheads of the Adams clasp. These arrowheads do not touch the adjoining teeth.

undercuts that are available for use as clasping surfaces are to be found buccally and lingually, mesially and distally on the deciduous molars, premolars, and molars, and mesially and distally on canines and incisors.

of the contact points and that the mesial and distal surfaces of the tooth below these points slope inwards quite sharply to the neck of the tooth, which is relatively narrow in a mesiodistal direction. Thus two further undercuts are available, one mesially, one distally, on this tooth. Not only are these undercuts more extensive than those on the buccal and lingual surfaces, but they begin much nearer to the occlusal surface of the tooth and are accessible when the tooth is at a much earlier stage of eruption than are the buccal and lingual undercuts, which do not come into view until the tooth is fully erupted. It will also be seen that the mesial and distal undercuts extend buccally and lingually and

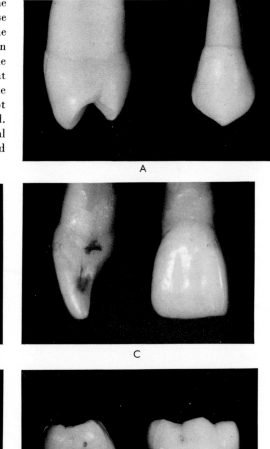

A

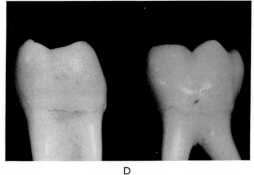

B

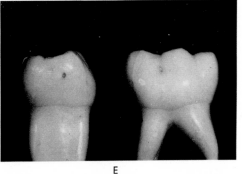

C

D

E

Fig. 52.—Mesial and buccal views of teeth showing the undercut areas bucco-lingually and mesiodistally. In all cases the mesiodistal undercuts are much nearer the occlusal or incisal surface.

A, Upper right first premolar; B, Upper right canine; C, Upper right central incisor; D, Lower left first permanent molar; E, Lower left second deciduous molar.

do not exist only in the median sagittal plane of the tooth (*Fig.* 51 C). They are, therefore, accessible from the buccal aspect for clasping purposes. The mesial and distal undercuts just described will be found to exist on all the other teeth, whether molars, deciduous or permanent, premolars, canines, or even incisors. (*Fig.* 52.)

It will be apparent that a clasp which is designed to make use of the mesial and distal undercuts of the teeth will be more effective for orthodontic purposes than any other if only because it will be effective in clasping semi-erupted teeth, and teeth in this state are found more often than not at the age at which patients usually undergo orthodontic treatment.

49

THE JACKSON CLASP

The Jackson clasp (V. H. Jackson, 1906) was expressly designed with a view to utilizing the mesial and distal undercuts, the wire of the clasp running around the cervical margin of the tooth buccally and then as far as possible interproximally, mesially and

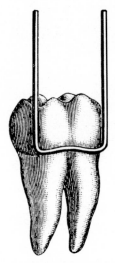

Fig. 53.—The Jackson clasp Note that the wire is carried mesially and distally into the undercut areas on the neck of the tooth. (*From V. H. Jackson in "Orthodontia and Orthopedia of the Face", Philadelphia, Lippincott, 1904.*)

distally at the gum margin (*Fig.* 53). While the value of the mesial and distal undercut was thus appreciated, it must be admitted that this form of clasp cannot use these retentive surfaces to the best advantages. If the buccal undercut is exposed by full eruption of the tooth, which is usually so where deciduous teeth are concerned, then a plain Jackson clasp, using this undercut alone and ignoring the mesial and distal undercuts, may be quite effective as a retention device (*Fig.* 54). This is especially so in certain instances where the deciduous molars have a marked ridge of enamel at the anatomical neck opposite the mesiobuccal root. The Jackson clasp will achieve very adequate retention over the sharp undercut available at this point. Fully erupted premolars and molars may also be clasped with the Jackson clasp using the

50

buccal and lingual undercuts only. Where teeth are only semi-erupted and where really firm and precise retention is required, a clasp using the mesial and distal undercuts is much to be preferred.

THE CROZAT CLASP

A clasp design suggested by Crozat (1920) is based on the plain crib form of clasp but makes

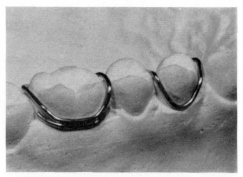

Fig. 54.—Right, the plain Jackson clasp. Left, the Crozat clasp, here made for illustration in stainless steel wire welded, but usually made in precious metal soldered. (*From Adams, C. P., "Removable Appliances Yesterday and Today", American Journal of Orthodontics, 55, 748–64, 1969. By kind permission.*)

use of mesial and distal undercuts by the addition of a short piece of wire which runs into the mesial and distal undercuts on the neck of the tooth (*Fig.* 54). The clasp is usually made in precious metal and the additional wire is soldered on.

ARROWHEAD CLASPS

The arrowhead type of clasp (A. M. Schwarz, 1956; J. A. C. Duyzings, 1954) makes use of the mesial and distal undercuts on the teeth. The central principle of action of these clasps is that an arrowhead, filed from a half-round clasp wire, or formed in a finer gauge of round stainless steel wire, is inserted between two teeth in approximal contact just below their contact points. In this way a very secure retention is achieved. It is possible, when a number of teeth are present in the arch and all in approximal contact, to place a number of arrowheads in the same buccal segment, so that two or three arrowheads may be used on each side of the same appliance.

The arrowhead type of clasp brought to removable appliance technique the great advantages of extreme security and reliability

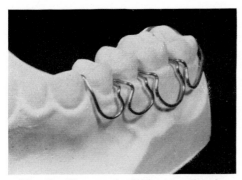

Fig. 55.—The arrowhead clasp attributed to Schwarz (1956). The arrowheads are formed by special pliers and are inserted into the spaces below the contact points between two teeth. A number of arrowheads may be embodied in one clasp as shown or only one or two may be used. (*From Adams, C. P., "Removable Appliances Yesterday and Today", American Journal of Orthodontics*, **55**, 748–64, 1969. *By kind permission.*)

of retention on semi-erupted teeth; features which could not always be achieved with the plain orthodontic clasp. The arrowhead clasp has, however, the drawbacks that specialized pliers are as a rule necessary for its construction, teeth in approximal contact are required for the development of the fullest retention, and there is a tendency in certain types of clasp for a large amount of wire to occupy the buccal sulcus, taking up space that could often better be used for bows and auxiliary springs, and occasionally interfering with and injuring the soft tissues of the sulcus and cheek. (*Fig.* 55.)

The Adams clasp or modified arrowhead clasp, sometimes referred to as the Liverpool clasp or Universal clasp, possesses all the advantages of the arrowhead type of clasp and has certain additional advantages of its own but has none of the disadvantages of the earlier type.

The Adams Clasp.—This clasp, which was first demonstrated in May, 1950, makes use of the mesial and distal undercuts of the teeth in the same way as the arrowhead type of clasp, but the Adams clasp is made to fit a single tooth, whether in approximal contact with the adjoining teeth or standing in isolation. The points or "arrowheads" of the modified form of clasp as described here do not fit beneath the contact points of two adjoining teeth. The advantages of this arrangement are that a single tooth may be clasped whether as part of a complete arch or not. The clasp also has the following advantages:—

1. The clasp is small, neat, and unobtrusive, and takes up a minimum of space in the buccal sulcus and in the baseplate.

2. The clasp may be used on any tooth, deciduous or permanent.

3. A tooth in a state of semi-eruption may be clasped.

4. The clasp is rigid and accurate, but resilient enough to give a firm grip for every retention purpose. A single short piece of wire is used, so giving adequate strength to resist the distorting and displacing forces of the occlusion during mastication.

5. No specialized pliers are required for constructing the clasp.

6. A number of variations of the clasp are available which extend the usefulness of the clasp in certain circumstances.

Construction of the Adams Clasp.—The clasp must be made of 0·7-mm. hard stainless steel wire for all teeth except canines for which 0·6-mm. wire is preferred. Adams universal pliers make the construction of the clasp particularly easy. The construction of the clasp should be done in a series of well-defined stages as follows:—

1. The plaster model of the tooth to be clasped should be carefully studied and it should be ascertained how far the tooth is erupted. If the tooth is only partly erupted it will be necessary to trim back the plaster representing the gum tissue, using a straight enamel chisel, so that the undercut mesially and distally on the tooth will be accessible to the clasp for fitting during the course of construction of the clasp (*Fig.* 56). When the finished appliance is placed in the mouth, the arrowheads of the clasp will then press back the interdental papillæ slightly and make

51

contact with definite undercuts on the tooth. It is most important not to carry the trimming of the plaster model to excess and to try to reach a part of the undercut too far below the gum margin. If the tooth is even half-erupted a very slight trimming back of the

when trimming the model and hence achieve accuracy of clasp adaptation.

If the tooth is fully erupted and there is actual gum recession beyond the anatomical neck of the tooth, as occurs sometimes in adults, very large and deep undercuts,

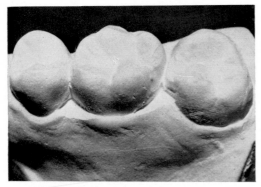

Fig. 56.—The trimming of the plaster model. This molar is fairly well erupted and the trimming shown indicates the average amount that requires to be done.

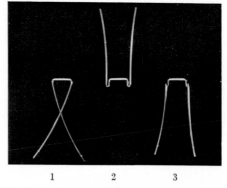

1   2   3

Fig. 57.—A summary of the stages in bending the Adams clasp.

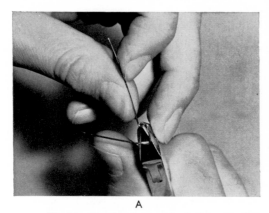

A

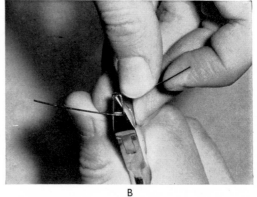

B

Fig. 58.—Forming the arrowhead, Stage 1 to Stage 2 (see Fig. 57). A, The first bend is at 90°. The clasp is then tilted in the pliers and held in the extreme tips of the beaks and, B, The tag is bent through a further 90°. Note that the thumb is used for bending and all possible fingers are used for support to steady the bending operation.

plaster representing the gum margin will be sufficient. It is also most important not to trim away any of the plaster that represents tooth tissue. If this is done, the clasp may be found to be too tight when placed in the mouth, a most undesirable fault. It is necessary to anticipate what will be the subgingival shape of the tooth and to reproduce that shape

mesially and distally, will be available for clasping purposes. It is then important to select as much of the undercut as may seem necessary for the purposes of the clasp and not to fit the clasp to the maximum clinically available undercut. The maximum available undercut on molar teeth, when there is gum recession, is actually too deep for clasping

52

purposes and a clasp that is made to fit into such a deep undercut will not be sufficiently elastic to spring over the most bulbous part of the tooth. In these circumstances it is

near the bend. The wire is *not* bent *around* the ends of the pliers but outside the tips of the beaks. The second arrowhead is formed in the same way.

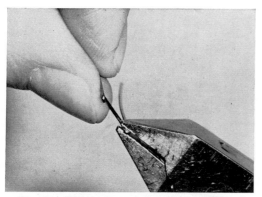

Fig. 59.—Tilting the arrowheads to correspond with the slope of the gum margin.

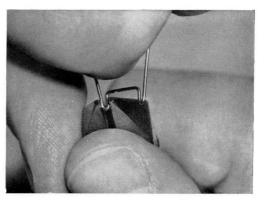

Fig. 60.—Squeezing the arrowheads. Note how thumbs and fingers concentrate on the area to control the application of force. The index finger of the left hand is put between the tags and exerts an outward pressure (i.e., to the left side of this picture) while the arrowhead is squeezed. This keeps the sides of the arrowhead parallel.

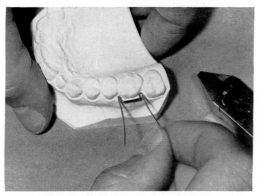

Fig. 61.—Trying the clasp on the tooth.

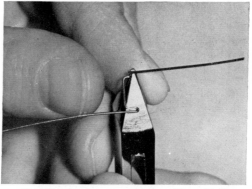

Fig. 62.—Bending over the tag. Note: (1) The arrowhead is only half-way into the pliers; (2) The arrowhead is held from *inside the clasp*; (3) The arrowhead is held by the extreme tip of the pliers; (4) The tag is bent outside the tip of the plier beak.

necessary to make the clasp touch the tooth only far enough below the level of the contact points to ensure adequate retention.

2. The stages in bending the wire for the clasp are shown in *Fig.* 57. Stage 1 will present no difficulty. The formation of the arrowhead is shown in *Fig.* 58 A, B. It should be noted that the arrowheads may be made quite long, shortness in itself is no advantage. The wire is first bent at a right angle (A) and the tag then tilted up and then, holding the wire firmly in the pliers, the tag is bent over through the remaining right angle using firm pressure with the thumb of the left hand on the wire

3. After the arrowheads are formed in the rough, it will usually be found that they slope both in the same direction when viewed end-on and one of them will have to be adjusted (*Fig.* 59) so that they will both conform to the slope of the gum margin of the tooth (*see also Fig.* 67). The arrowheads are

then squeezed up to the correct degree of narrowness (*Fig.* 60). While this is being done, a firm outward pressure is maintained on the tag to ensure that the sides of the arrowhead remain parallel.

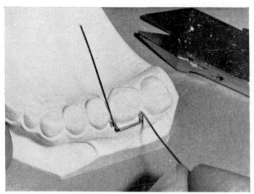

Fig. 63.—Trying the tag for alinement and angular position of the bridge.

4. The clasp is then tried on the tooth to see that the tips of the arrowheads are the correct distance apart (*Fig.* 61). There is considerable latitude in the distance between the points of the arrowheads, which will prove satisfactory when fitting these clasps to molars and canines. If the clasp errs in the direction of being too wide in span, however, it is better to discard it and make a narrower clasp. If the arrowheads are too far apart there will be a tendency for them to disappear in between the teeth altogether and the bridge between the arrowheads may be found to lie against the buccal surface of the tooth. Also too wide a clasp will show a tendency for the arrowheads to impinge on the adjoining teeth, which will prevent the clasp from acting properly on the tooth which is being clasped.

It is particularly important when clasping premolars to realize that the necks of these teeth are very narrow and to avoid making the clasp too wide to fit properly.

5. When the width and fit of the clasp are considered satisfactory, the tags are turned over and brought across the contact points and on to the lingual side of the dental arch for embedding in the baseplate (Stage 2 to Stage 3; *Fig.* 57). This bend must be made

sharply and accurately and must not be allowed to project beyond the bridge of the clasp and hence, later on, into the soft tissues of the cheek. The bend is made by grasping the arrowhead from the inside of the

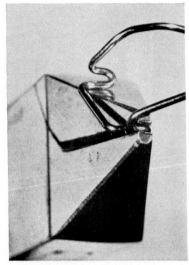

Fig. 64.—Bending over the tag (second tag). Note that the tag is bent outside the tip of the plier beak and not over the tip of the beak.

clasp (*Fig.* 62) and only holding half of the arrowhead at the very tip of the pliers. The wire is then bent outside the tip of the pliers and not around the end of the beak. The method advocated makes it possible to make a really sharp bend at this point. The clasp is again tried on the tooth for alinement of the tag, inclination of the arrowheads, and position of the bridge (*Fig.* 63), and any necessary adjustments are made. When this stage is satisfactory, the tag is finished off and the second tag then bent up and finished (*Fig.* 64; *see also Fig.* 68).

The tags need not be finished off in a complicated manner; if the end of the tag is turned down at right angles for a distance of 1·5–2 mm., this will ensure positive and secure anchorage of the tag in the baseplate material. Tags should be of a harmonious length; excessively long tags divide up the baseplate too much and use up space in the baseplate which may be needed for the embedding of other wires. Tags, on the other hand, should not be made very short unless lack of space in the baseplate leaves no alternative.

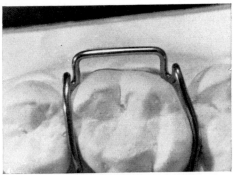

Fig. 65.

a. The arrowheads must not impinge on the adjoining teeth.

b. The arrowheads must be squeezed up to an appropriate narrowness *but not so far that the wire becomes damaged at the bend at the tip of the arrowhead.*

c. The arrowheads are not made as short as is possible. Extreme shortness is not of itself a virtue. The arrowheads should be made reasonably long ; this facilitates construction and has the effect also of keeping the bridge away from the tooth and from the soft tissue adjoining the cervical margin.

d. It has been found that the practice of adjusting the width between the arrowheads by bending the bridge between them should be avoided. The bridge between the arrowheads should be straight and the arrowheads themselves parallel to one another.

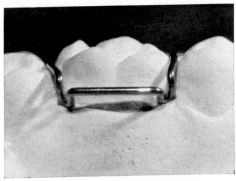

Fig. 67.—The arrowheads are sloped to follow the line of the gum margin.

When designing an appliance, ensure always that only one tag is brought over the embrasure between any two teeth. Only if the teeth are sufficiently spaced and there is freedom from the bite of the opposing dental arch may this rule be broken.

Essential Features of the Adams Clasp.— These are illustrated and summarized in *Figs.* 65–68 and their captions.

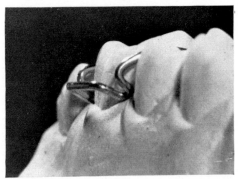

Fig. 66.

a. The bridge between the arrowheads should project and be arranged midway between the buccal surface of the tooth and the adjoining gingival tissue, so avoiding contact with either. If the bridge lies near the gum margin, when the clasp is tightened the bridge will come down on the soft tissue causing pain and irritation.

b. The point at which the wire bends from the arrowhead to cross over the contact point should not project beyond the bridge but should be well inside it.

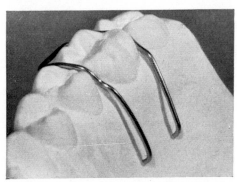

Fig. 68.—The tags should cross the contact points lying as closely as possible against the teeth and should be fitted into the lingual embrasure. The ends of the tags are turned down sharply to support the tag with a definite space between it and the soft tissue so that the baseplate material will flow completely around the tag and hold it firmly. This feature also has the effect of stabilizing the clasp during the laboratory packing process.

Adjusting the Adams Clasp.—When the appliance has been processed, polished, and is placed in the mouth, the arrowheads of the clasps should just make contact with the teeth but should not grip to any noticeable degree.

55

The accuracy of fit of the baseplate and of the positioning of springs and archwires, with all these metal parts quite passive, is checked at this stage.

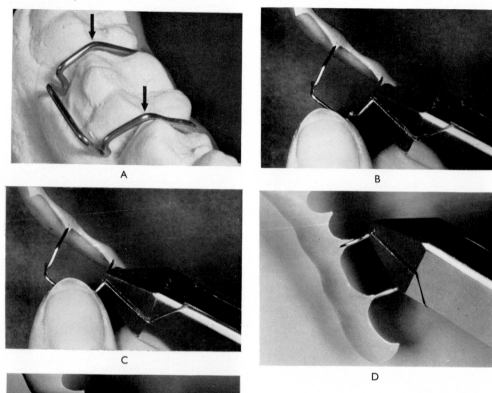

If all is well, finger springs are cut off and the free ends turned into loops and the points of application of the springs are adjusted without activating the springs. The fit and position of heavy bows are adjusted if necessary and any fine apron springs required are attached,

formed and adjusted for position on the teeth.

The clasps should then be adjusted to grip the teeth sufficiently by bending the tags a

Fig. 69.—Adjusting the Adams clasp. When the appliance is first inserted, the clasp should not be tight. **A**, The clasp is tightened by bending the tags just where they cross the outer part of the embrasure, as shown by the arrows. Bending the tag at any point nearer to the baseplate will only cause the tag to ride up on the embrasure. The bend is made by grasping the tag as shown in **B, C** and pressing the arrowhead slightly towards the baseplate with the thumb. Alternatively, if the outer wire is short and difficult to bend, this outer wire may be grasped in the pliers and the inner part of the tag used to make the bend, taking care to make the bend only at the spot shown by the arrow, **D, E.**

little, just buccally to the point where they cross the contact points of the teeth. This adjustment is most easily made with Adams universal pliers although any fine-beaked pliers may be used. To make the adjustment, the tag is gripped firmly and bent slightly. Both tags on any clasp should always be adjusted. (*Fig.* 69.)

Over-tightening of the clasp should be avoided as being unnecessary and making the removal of the appliance unduly difficult for the patient.

Modifications of the Adams Clasp.—From time to time modifications of the Adams clasp are suggested as being required to overcome alleged disadvantages in the clasp or as improvements on the original design. In the twenty years since this clasp was introduced, no change in its principle of action, form, or construction has been found necessary. Drawbacks or disadvantages that are sometimes suggested can invariably be traced to faulty understanding of the principles underlying the design of the clasp or simply to failure to construct the clasp to the proper outline.

The Preformed Adams Clasp.—Adams clasps, preformed to Stage 3 (*Fig.* 57), are now to be obtained.* The use of these parts eliminates three stages in clasp bending, with a corresponding saving of time, and there is the further advantage that the clasps are uniform and accurate in configuration. A wide range of sizes is available in the recommended gauges of wire.

To fit a preformed Adams clasp it is only necessary to trim the gingival margin of the working model (*Fig.* 56), and to fit the clasp as in *Fig.* 63, with the difference that both tags have been bent up preparatory to fitting them over the embrasures between the teeth. Before fitting the clasp, the parallelism of the arrowheads and the tilting to correspond with the curve of the gum margin should be checked and if necessary adjusted (*Figs.* 65, 67).

---

* The preformed Adams clasp. Manufactured by the Unitek Corporation, Monrovia, California.

CHAPTER VI

VARIATIONS OF THE ADAMS CLASP

THE Adams clasp can be used to clasp any tooth, deciduous or permanent, and is efficient in the retention of all types of removable appliance.

From time to time, however, variations of the design, and extensions of the use of the clasp have been suggested and tried out. The following variations will be found to be particularly effective.

Canines and Deciduous Molars.—*Figs.* 70 and 71 show the construction of the clasp for deciduous molars and canines. For canines, 0·6-mm. wire is best, as it is sufficiently strong and can be well fitted into the groove between the canine and the adjoining teeth on the lingual side (*Fig.* 72), so avoiding the bite of the lower incisors. For deciduous molars 0·7-mm. wire is used. The clasp must be very carefully made on account of the shallowness of the crowns of these teeth, otherwise the tags of the clasps may not lie closely enough in the embrasure between the marginal ridges, and may interfere unnecessarily with the occlusion.

Rotated Teeth.—If the tooth to be clasped is rotated (*Fig.* 73), the clasp is applied exactly as if the tooth were in normal position. That

is to say, the bridge between the arrowheads is kept parallel to the general line of the arch and is not rotated so as to remain parallel to the buccal surface of the tooth. The reasons for

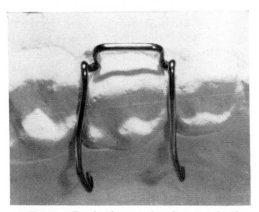

Fig. 70.—For deciduous molars do not make the clasp too wide, keep tags well down on the embrasures.

this are, firstly, while one undercut of the tooth has rotated out of sight and reach, the other has become more accessible and an excellent grip can be obtained on it with one arrowhead, while the other arrowhead, if not

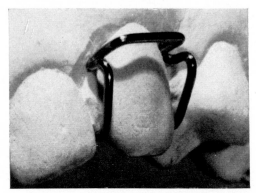 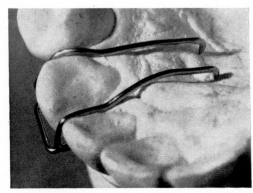

Figs. 71, 72.—For canines use 0·6-mm. wire and fit the tags well down between the teeth on the lingual side.

perhaps having an undercut to grip, still impinges on the tooth and stabilizes the clasp as a whole. Secondly, to rotate the clasp

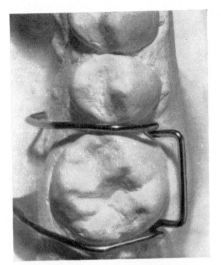

Fig. 73.—When clasping a rotated tooth keep the bridge parallel to the line of the arch.

involves the risk of bringing one arrowhead into contact with the tooth adjoining.

Traction Hooks.—Intermaxillary traction hooks may be either incorporated in the

merits of strength and ease of construction, and requires no welding or soldering. *Fig. 75* is the same hook on an upper first premolar. If the sulcus is shallow behind and below a lower tooth, as sometimes happens with a lower first permanent molar, it is not feasible to use this form of hook, as it is inclined to project into the soft tissue where it is reflected from the alveolar process at the bottom of the sulcus.

The alternatives are shown in *Fig. 76*, a simple turn in the bridge over or through which the elastic is looped, or the hook in *Fig. 77* A, which may be soldered or welded using 0·7-mm. soft wire. The free end of this hook should be turned in under the bridge of the clasp (*Fig. 77* B) to avoid irritating the soft tissue of the cheek.

Often, in place of an upper traction hook, it is convenient to loop the elastic over the bridge of a plain clasp before the plate is inserted and the other end of the elastic is hooked in the ordinary way on to a hook on the lower clasp.

The Single Arrowhead.—Where the last tooth in the lower arch is semi-erupted, as often occurs with a first permanent molar at 6 to 7 years of age, or a second permanent

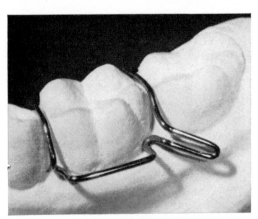

Fig. 74.—The standard lower posterior traction hook. Very strong, simple to construct.

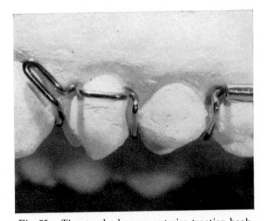

Fig. 75.—The standard upper anterior traction hook.

bending of the clasp or else welded or soldered to the normal type of clasp later on. *Fig.* 74 shows the standard traction hook incorporated in the bending of the clasp. This has the

molar at 11 or 12 years of age, the distal undercut is not accessible, and on that account the distal arrowhead is omitted. The mesial arrowhead, however, in conjunction with a

59

clasp on a premolar farther forward, provides valuable retention (*Fig.* 78).

The Accessory Arrowhead.—Where utmost retention is required and two teeth on one contact with one another must be condemned. Such clasps cannot be fully effective, or easily adjusted, and it is rarely desirable to have two tags passing over the same contact point.

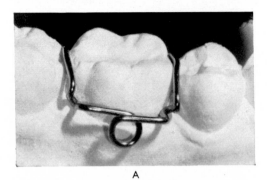

A

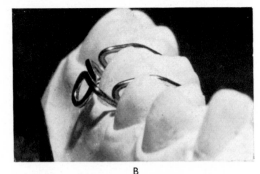

B

Fig. 76.—The loop hook for a shallow sulcus. No welding or soldering required.

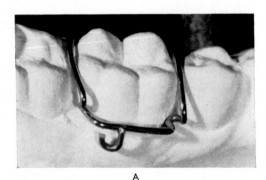

A

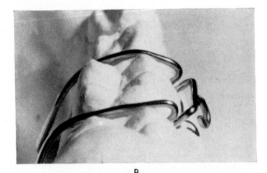

B

Fig. 77.—The welded or soldered hook. Can be put on if hooks have been overlooked in the construction of the plate.

side separated from one another by a space or by a third tooth are not available, two adjoining teeth may be clasped using the accessory arrowhead. *Figs.* 79 and 80 show this clasp, constructed for use on $\overline{6E|}$ in *Fig.* 79 and for $|56$ in *Fig.* 80, where it was desired to have very firm retention of the plate and to move $|4$. The free tag of the accessory arrowhead is welded or soldered to the bridge of the main arrowhead after the plate is processed. Before this soldering or welding is done, the appliance should be tried in and the accessory arrowhead should be checked for accuracy of fit.

The practice of putting modified arrowhead clasps on two adjoining teeth which are in

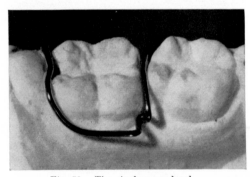

Fig. 78.—The single arrowhead.

Tubes.—It is common practice to-day to use tubes on Adams clasps either on molars for free-sliding arches used in the retraction of

60

upper incisors with intermaxillary or extra-oral traction, or on premolars for the attachment of a night-time extra-oral appliance to an intermaxillary traction plate.

margin or with the occlusion as the case may be. If attached laterally, it may project too far into the cheek and cause irritation. The needs of each case must be carefully studied and the placing of the tube decided on with these difficulties in mind. (*See Figs.* 238–241.)

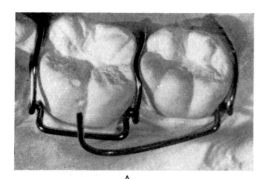

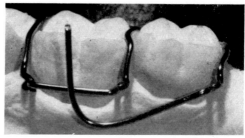

Fig. 79.—The accessory arrowhead during construction.

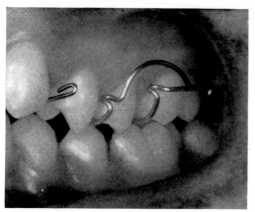

Fig. 80.—The accessory arrowhead in the mouth.

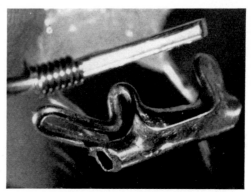

Fig. 81.—Tube on an upper first premolar showing the end of the extra-oral attachment which plugs into the tube. Note Trevor Johnson friction-fit stop.

These tubes are easily attached by free-hand soldering after the plate has been processed.

If the plate is replaced on the model on which it was waxed up and processed and a long length of tubing is used, orientation of the tubing is greatly facilitated. The actual length of tubing required is then cut free and trimmed down to size and smoothed (*Figs.* 81, 82). The baseplate material should be kept cool by covering it with a wet napkin during soldering. The tube may be attached to the bridge of the clasp laterally or directly above or below. If attached directly above or below, the tube is liable to interfere with the gum

Variation in Gauge of Wire.—Some operators have found that in their hands the clasps work better if made in certain circumstances in gauges of wire thinner or thicker than 0·7 mm. The writer has found that 0·7-mm. wire satisfies all requirements for molars, premolars, and deciduous molars. 0·6-mm. wire has been found most suitable for canines.

Fractures of the Clasp.—There are two sharp bends in the clasp, both in the neighbourhood of the arrowhead. If these bends are made once during construction of the clasp, as they should be, and are not bent and re-bent, they will not break in use. It does happen occasionally, however, that a clasp will fracture at one or other of these bends owing to over-stressing of the wire during construction of the clasp. If the wire is cleaned with a cuttlefish disk and the ends accurately opposed with the wire made passive, the lumen of the loop may be filled with solder, so effecting a rapid repair (*Fig.* 83). The base-plate adjoining the clasp should be wrapped in a damp napkin for protection during soldering.

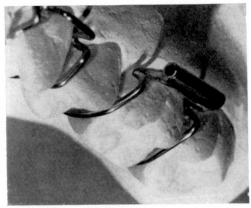

Fig. 82.—Tube on molar clasp for free-sliding buccal arch.

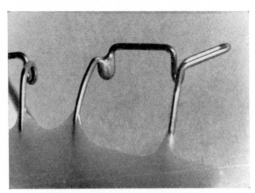

Fig. 83.—Soldered repair of arrowhead.

CHAPTER VII

LABIO- AND BUCCO-LINGUAL
MOVEMENT OF TEETH

LABIO- and bucco-lingual movement is, as a rule, a very straightforward tooth movement with removable appliances, for the reason that a purely inclining movement produces a satisfactory effect. The position of the apices of the teeth in a bucco-lingual direction is to a great extent determined by skeletal development, and it is not often necessary to alter the position of the apices of the teeth in the basal bone in this particular direction. Pure inclination of the teeth in a bucco-lingual direction for the most part, therefore, generally suffices.

PROCLINATION OF UPPER INCISORS

Perhaps the most commonly performed movement of this kind is the proclination of a single upper incisor over the bite. There are very many variations in the details of cases of this kind, from the early case in which the erupting central incisor, with adequate space in the arch, is barely caught behind the bite of the lower incisors, to the older case in which all the deciduous teeth have been shed, the premolars are up, and a single upper incisor has been caught deeply behind the bite of the lower incisors, possibly with barely enough room for it in the arch. In both cases the factors militating against movement of the misplaced tooth into line are: the incisal overlap; the possibility of having to move a tooth into a space that is too small for it; the possible effect of lip pressure on the movement of the misplaced tooth; and the speed of reaction of the bone to pressure.

The incisor overlap will vary greatly from case to case, but if it is anything more than very slight in amount, precautions should be taken to free the occlusion before attempting to move the misplaced tooth. If a locked incisor is pushed labially, without freeing the occlusion, the intermittent impact of occlusion against a steady forward pressure on the

tooth soon produces marked loosening of the tooth and usually periodontal pain. It is, therefore, advisable to free the interlock of the upper and lower incisors by means of bite planes. Bite planes may be used either in the molar region or in the incisor region. The choice of site for the bite planes will depend on the details of the occlusion and the degree

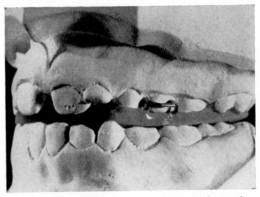

Fig. 84.—The bite plane must be just high enough to clear the bite of the front teeth and must be arranged so that all the lower teeth bite against it.

of overbite. For instance, in a case with very slight overbite an anterior bite plane will have a tendency to reduce the overbite further, which would be undesirable. Furthermore, in a case in which all the upper incisors are behind the bite an incisal bite plane would not be feasible at all and it would be necessary in such a case to use bite planes in the molar region.

Before attempting to move an incisor forward over the bite it should be ascertained that there is in fact room for it in the arch. This point is sometimes overlooked, and it is difficult or impossible to push a tooth into a space that is too small for it.

A single upper incisor locked behind the bite does not as a rule present much difficulty

63

in treatment. In the young patient the malocclusion is usually found at an early stage when there is very little incisor overbite. In most of these cases it is not feasible to use an anterior bite plane as there is a mixture of deciduous

made as long as possible within the limits imposed by the dental arch and should be provided with a guard or guide which has the dual purpose of holding the spring down to the point at which it is desired to press on the

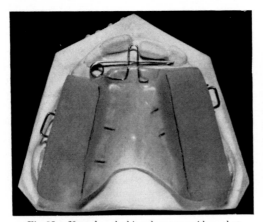

Fig. 85.—Note that the bite planes are wide so that the lower teeth have a sufficient area to bite over. The spring is of 0·5-mm. wire.

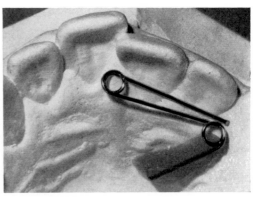

Fig. 86.—Double cantilever spring. This may be used on two or more teeth. Normally of 0·5-mm. wire. If four teeth are being moved, 0·6-mm. wire may be used.

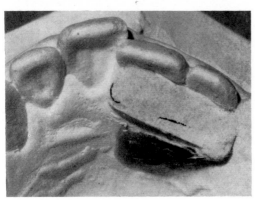

Fig. 87.—The double cantilever spring plastered in.

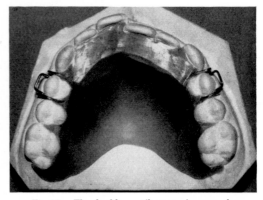

Fig. 88.—The double cantilever spring waxed up. Note that the anterior bite plane is *flat* and has a definite posterior edge, arranged so far back that the lower incisors cannot bite behind it.

and permanent teeth in this region, some loose and some hardly erupted. It is better to use posterior bite planes which must be contoured so that the opposing dental arch bites evenly against it, each tooth carrying a part of the occlusal stress. The patient can then eat with the plate in position (*Figs.* 84, 85).

A single tooth is most easily moved across the bite with a single cantilever spring with a coil at the point of attachment to increase the range of action (*Fig.* 85). The spring should be

tooth, and also to protect the spring to some extent against the effects of masticating a mouthful of food. This appliance has the advantages that the spring is easy to find and compress with the finger and the appliance can be inserted by the youngest patient. The spring will operate for periods of up to one month, depending on the rate at which the tooth moves.

For the patient in whom the overbite is greater than normal it is often better to use an anterior bite plane. The construction and use of the spring are then complicated by the necessity to box it in with an acrylic bite plane.

In cases in which more than one tooth is to be moved over the bite, it is best to use the double cantilever spring (*Fig.* 86). This spring is simple and positive in its action; it is, however, difficult to control with a wire guard and is usually boxed in instead (*Figs.* 87, 88). A wire guard is not efficient unless it controls the spring over its effective range of action. In *Fig.* 86 it can be seen that a wire guard cannot be arranged over the space that the spring will move into as the teeth are already occupying this space. In this form the double cantilever spring may be used to procline two, three, or four incisors over the bite, the overlap of the incisors being temporarily removed by means of posterior bite planes if necessary.

Where two or more upper incisors are to be proclined a conventional expansion screw may be used to produce the movement. The inclusion of a screw in an upper baseplate just behind the incisors increases the bulk of the appliance somewhat, but careful construction will minimize any inconvenience. If an anterior bite plane is used, the screw can usually be incorporated in the bulk of the bite plane (*Fig.* 89). Posterior bite planes may, of course, be used.

A point that should be borne in mind is that the lingual surface of the upper incisors is not vertical near the cervical margin, but slopes towards the cingulum. A horizontal pressure on this surface produces a vertical component that tends to shorten or depress the tooth. It should be remembered, therefore, when proclining upper incisors that have a very slight overbite with the lowers, that the pressure required to procline them may shorten them so that the overbite disappears altogether. This possibility should always be anticipated.

PROCLINATION OF LOWER INCISORS

Two or more lower incisors may be proclined with a double cantilever spring, but a rather

more effective method of producing this movement is by means of a lingual arch to which are attached apron springs (*Fig.* 90). The lingual arch is made of 1·25-mm. hard wire and the auxiliary spring of 0·3-mm. hard wire.

The end of the spring wire is anchored to the baseplate by means of a steel tape loop. This tape attachment is made of soft stainless

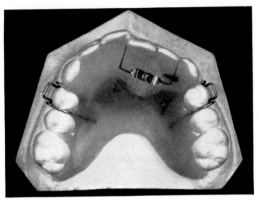

Fig. 89.—Proclination of two incisors by means of a screw. Three or four incisors may equally well be moved in this way. The small black arrow reminds the patient which way to turn the screw.

steel tape approximately 2·5 mm. × 0.15 mm. The tape is first formed on a wire blank (*Fig.* 91) and embedded in the wax at the edge of the plate (*Fig.* 92), and waxed right up to the loop containing the wire. This wire holds the tape in position during the packing and processing operations and when the plate is finished the wire is pulled out. A fresh wire is formed into a loop at one end and pulled in until the loop jams.

The short end of the wire is turned back and ground off, the long end is used to form the spring (*Fig.* 93). Only three coils are wound on the archwire as it is of substantial gauge and the coils are, therefore, fairly large. The spring may be made to act on three teeth as shown, or on two or even on one. As an alternative to the tape attachment, the apron spring may be attached to the arch at any point that may be desired by means of electro-welding. This has the advantage that the spring may be fixed near the centre of the arch if only a central incisor is to be moved and a neater arrangement of the spring results. Soldering an apron spring to such a thick wire is not satisfactory as the rather large amount of heat required may travel as far as

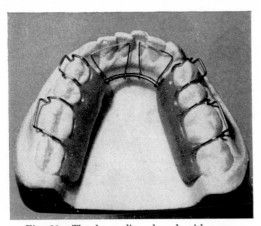

Fig. 90.—The lower lingual arch with apron springs.

It is important in this type of appliance to see that the plate is firmly held down anteriorly. It is, therefore, usual to put clasps on

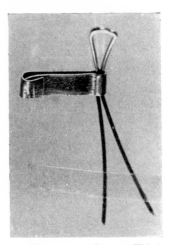

Fig. 91.—The tape attachment. This is pinched up tight around the wire blank.

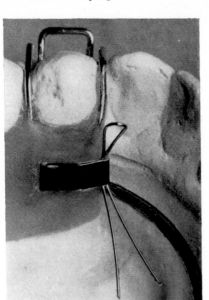

Fig. 92.—The tape attachment placed in the edge of the plate, before covering in with wax.

the acrylic baseplate and lead to damage of the acrylic. Also soldering involves risk of annealing the arch, which would be most undesirable as the strength of the plate depends mostly on the strength of this arch.

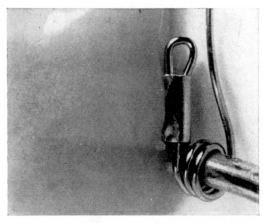

Fig. 93.—The completed attachment with the spring wire in position. The buried part of the tape can be faintly seen through the acrylic.

the first premolars as well as clasps farther back.

In mixed dentitions it may not be possible to clasp the lower first molar and as an alternative the auxiliary arrowhead clasp may be used. Clasps posteriorly, however, are not as a rule sufficient as there is a strong tendency for the appliance to rise at the front under the influence of the reaction of the springs.

BUCCAL MOVEMENT OF MOLARS AND PREMOLARS

The buccal movement of molars and premolars can also best be carried out with cantilever springs in one form or another. The main difficulty usually is to provide retention for the plate on the side on which springs are being placed, as the springs take up much space and the choice of teeth for clasping is, therefore, limited.

In *Figs.* 94, 95 the premolar is being moved buccally and it should be noted that the following features are incorporated in the spring:—

1. It is of adequate length.

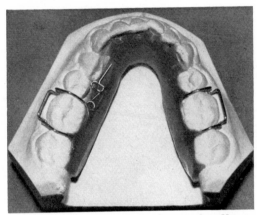

Fig. 94.—Buccal movement of a premolar. Note that anchorage is achieved from 765432|6. Spring of 0·5-mm. wire.

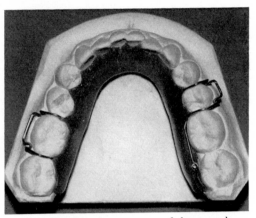

Fig. 96.—Buccal movement of lower molar. Anchorage from 5|34567. Spring of 0·5-mm. wire wound on 1·0-mm. support.

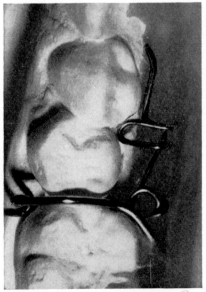

Fig. 95.—Buccal movement of premolar. Detail of the spring. The tip of the spring has been turned in to avoid catching the tongue.

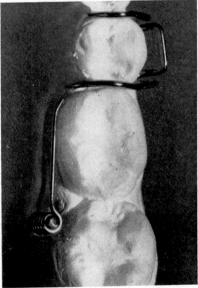

Fig. 97.—Detail of spring in *Fig.* 96. The coils of the spring must be plastered and waxed in to protect the tongue.

2. A guard and guide is provided which follows the spring right through its effective range of action.

It has been necessary in this instance to crank the spring so that it will not impinge on the second premolar. The cranking also makes

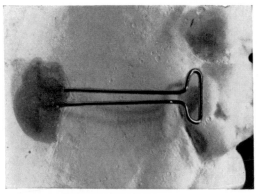

Fig. 98.—Buccal movement of upper molar. The spring is of 0·5-mm. wire attached about two-thirds of the way down towards the middle line of the palate from the gingival margin.

the guard for the spring more effective by increasing the distance over which it keeps the spring under control.

In the molar region in the lower arch there is often little room to make a cantilever spring with an effective range of action. The limitations imposed by lack of space may be overcome by winding a spring with four or five coils. A very long range of action may thus be achieved without having to make the arm of the spring too long. A support is made of wire 1·0 mm. thick and a spring is wound on it of 0·5-mm. wire (*Figs.* 2, 96, 97). It is necessary to finish off the top of the support very smoothly and to box in the whole spring to protect the tongue, which may otherwise become rubbed by the spring and the top of the support. It will be noticed that no guide is provided for this spring. It is a difficult position in which to place a guide and in any case it is found that the support on which the spring is wound has a stabilizing effect on the arm of the spring and that a guide can be dispensed with.

The buccal movement of teeth in the upper arch is carried out in the same way as for

teeth in the lower arch. The spring shown in *Fig.* 95 does not adapt itself well to use in the upper arch, but the large expanse of palate lends itself to the use of a spring of the type shown in *Figs.* 98, 99, which is useful for buccal movement of molars. This spring is formed of

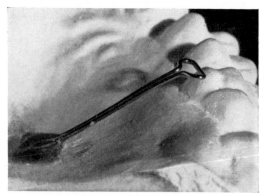

Fig. 99.—The spring shown in *Fig.* 98 is applied to the tooth near the occlusal surface and is clear of the palate.

0·5-mm. wire and is not made with a coil, as it is long enough to have an effective range of action without. The end which bears on the tooth is applied as near the coronal surface as possible so that as the tooth moves buccally the spring will slide down the tooth to a point near the gum margin. This spring has the great advantage that it does not need to be compressed by the patient while inserting the plate, the action of the appliance being quite automatic. After the spring is constructed, it must be plastered in and covered over by the baseplate. It then lies in a compartment between the plate and the palate and is activated by lifting slightly away from the baseplate.

RETROCLINATION OF UPPER INCISORS

The retroclination of upper incisors is a frequently required tooth movement in orthodontic treatment. Formerly this movement was carried out with a labial arch coming from somewhere towards the back of the mouth with a U-loop on either side to permit adjustment of the arch and the application of pressure to the front teeth, the reaction being distributed to the teeth in the buccal segments.

The complaint was frequently made that this treatment as frequently produced a forward movement of the buccal segments as it did a retroclination of the upper incisors. There is no doubt that this form of appliance has the

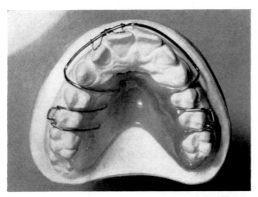

Fig. 100.—Retroclination of upper incisors. Note that the baseplate embraces every possible tooth for purposes of anchorage. The high labial bow stands just clear of the alveolus.

serious disadvantage that the active part, the labial bow, is very rigid and therefore it can only have a very short range of action. It also follows that over this short range of action

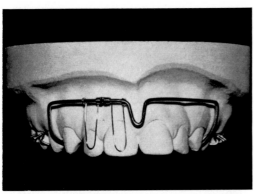

Fig. 101.—High labial bow. Note that it is straight and level. V loop is to avoid injury to frænum. The sharp right angles at the outer ends make it possible to attach spring wire, if preferred, by entangling it about this angle.

such a bow must exert a very high pressure. It is thus quite possible that when this appliance is used to retract upper incisors, the pressure in these teeth is so high that the periodontal blood-vessels are occluded and the

normal process of resorption and deposition of bone cannot proceed and the teeth cannot move. The reaction of the pressure, however, being distributed over the larger teeth in the buccal segments is reduced in terms of grammes

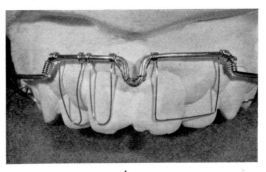

A

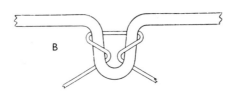

B

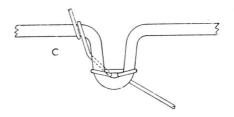

C

Fig. 102.—Attachment of apron springs by wrapping. A, The springs which are acting on $\underline{1|12}$ are formed from one piece of wire 0·3 mm. thick. The archwire is 1·0 mm. thick. B, The spring wire is first looped around the lowest part of the V in the arch and pulled tight. C, The coils of the springs are then wound. This preserves the function of the V which is to avoid injury to the frænum. The apron spring on $|12$ has an additional set of active coils at its outer or distal end.

per square millimetre of root area to a pressure that produces the normal process of bone resorption and forward movement of the buccal segments takes place.

What is required when retroclining front teeth, as is necessary when moving teeth in any other part of the mouth, is a continual gentle pressure over an adequate distance. This may be achieved by using springs of fine

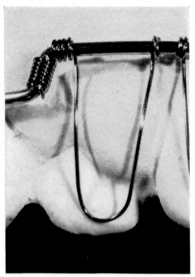

Fig. 103.—Attaching a single apron spring by wrapping. The spring wire is wrapped tightly around the vertical part of a sharp right angle in the archwire. The active coils are then wound on the horizontal part.

rule two clasps are sufficient to retain the plate in position. The plate must of course be cut away from the lingual surfaces of the front teeth. The

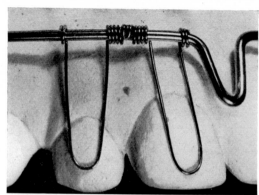

Fig. 104.—Attachment of apron springs by soldering.

high labial arch of 1·0-mm. or 0·9-mm. hard wire is made to cross the embrasure between the teeth in the buccal segments as closely as possible, so as not to interfere with the occlusion, and is made to run horizontally across the front of the mouth so as to provide an accurate point of attachment for the springs (*Fig.* 101). Usually it is necessary to place a V-loop centrally in the arch to accommodate

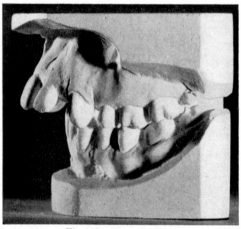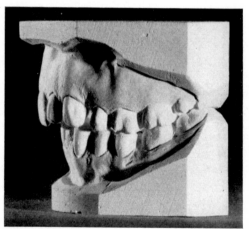

Fig. 105.—Retroclination of upper incisors without bringing buccal segments forward. Patient aged 22.

gauge attached to a heavy arch which acts as an extension of the baseplate. In practice the baseplate must be made to embrace as many as possible of the teeth in the buccal segments in order to provide anchorage (*Fig.* 100). As a

the frænum labii. The arch must not lie too high in the sulcus or stand too far away from the alveolus or it will irritate the lip.

The springs are made of 0·3-mm. wire attached to the arch by welding, soldering,

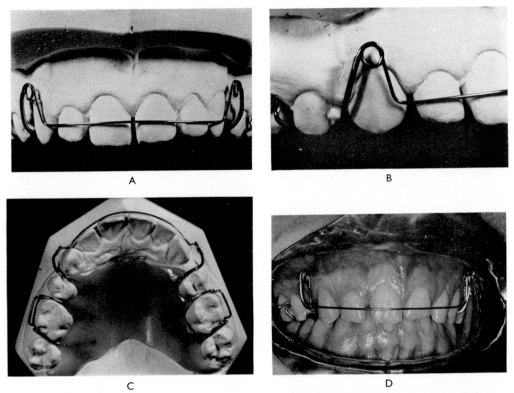

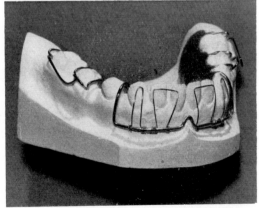

Fig. 106.—An appliance for retracting the teeth of the upper labial segment *en bloc* suggested by Roberts (1956). **A**, A labial apron of 0·5-mm. wire, with a coil spring at either side, rests about the middle of the incisor teeth or a little below. **B**. The apron wire from the coils to the baseplate is sheathed in annealed stainless steel tubing. **C**, Occlusal view. **D**, The incisors, formerly proclined and spaced, were retroclined with the appliance shown.

or by winding firmly around an angle in the arch. The neatest way is by soldering, which takes up the least space on the arch and provides a positive and permanent attachment (*Figs*. 104, 236, 237). The welding method, using tape, is also positive and permanent, but requires the necessary special equipment. (*See Fig.* 233.)

Where soldering or welding facilities are not available, springs may be attached by wrapping several turns of the spring wire tightly around an angle or kink in the supporting arch. Sharp angles must be made in the archwire and the spring wire must be wound very tightly so that a firm attachment, free from backlash, is achieved. The best method is to form a sharp angle of, at most, 90° and to wrap the spring wire at either side of this angle. The final turns of wire usually form the active coils of the spring. If an even sharper

Fig. 107.—Low labial bow and apron springs for retroclination of lower incisors and canines. Auxiliary springs of 0·3-mm. wire.

71

bend is available in the archwire, the spring may be actually tied into this kink and pulled tight with pliers. (*Figs.* 102, 103.)

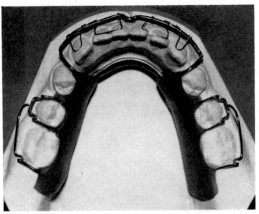

Fig. 108.—Retroclination of lower labial segment. The lingual arch is well clear of the alveolar process. Note apron arrowhead clasps to incorporate the first molars in the anchorage segment.

a U loop and coil at either side. The arms of the U loops from the coils right through into the baseplate material are reinforced with

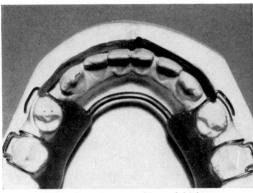

Fig. 109.—Retroclination of lower labial segment. The elastics exert a very suitable pressure. This appliance is not effective on the upper arch because it is usually more acutely curved and the elastic is not easily kept in position.

After the spring wire is attached to the arch, four coils at least should be wound and then the arm of the spring made as shown, in the form of a U or V of wire, the free end being turned around the arch. If the spring wire is doubled and attached at the point of bending two springs may be wound side by side (*Fig.* 104). In this way a series of independent springs may be constructed to act on a row of teeth. When retroclining upper incisors some operators prefer to construct a single apron spring running from side to side and pressing on all the incisors simultaneously. This type of spring is suitable when it is not necessary to have independent control over the teeth that are being moved.

The appliance just described has the outstanding advantage that it produces an absolutely controlled pressure on the front teeth so that if necessary the total pressure can be kept low enough to avoid any forward movement of the buccal segments (*Fig.* 105).

Roberts (1956) has suggested an apron type of spring, for the lingual movement of the teeth in the upper labial segment, in which the high labial bow is not required. The apron spring is made in hard wire 0·5 mm. thick with

tubing. The teeth in the labial segment must be retracted in unison and it may not be possible to produce special effects on individual teeth, but the appliance is efficient and unobtrusive and has a very good range of action. (*Fig.* 106.)

RETROCLINATION OF LOWER INCISORS

The same kind of appliance may be used to retrocline lower incisors, and all the previously mentioned considerations apply again (*Fig.* 107). In the lower arch, there being no palatal part of the plate, it must be made thick enough anteriorly to allow trimming to be done from the thickness of the plate to let the lower incisors retrocline. Otherwise a lingual bar may be used leaving space between the bar and the gingival tissue (*Fig.* 108). Lower incisors may also be retroclined by means of the appliance illustrated in *Fig.* 109. An elastic is looped from side to side across the labial surfaces of the lower incisors. If one elastic is too short two may be looped end to end and different combinations tried until an appropriate tension is achieved. It will be found that the patient needs to control the position of the elastic to some extent in a vertical direction as there will be a tendency for it to slip over the incisal edges of the teeth. This tendency can be reduced by placing the elastic towards the gingival margin rather than near the incisal edges of the teeth, and, in cases where the incisors and canines are arranged in a marked curve, by bringing the hooks a little farther forward.

LINGUAL MOVEMENT OF CANINES, PREMOLARS, AND MOLARS

The lingual movement of canines and teeth in the buccal segments can be done with heavy arches and springs of the kind that have just been described, but as a rule it is more satisfactory to use self-supporting springs because they are simpler in construction and use and except in the upper arch there is not enough room in the sulcus for an effective high

the spring illustrated in *Fig.* 110. It will be argued that in such a spring the coil does not lie in the plane of action of the free end.

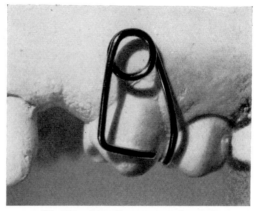

Fig. 110.—Lingual movement of premolar.

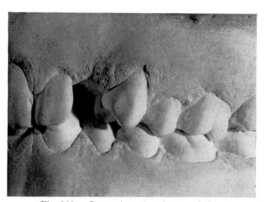
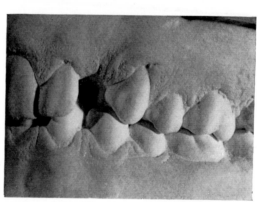

Fig. 111.—Correction of occlusion of |4 by lingual movement of |4 and buccal movement of |4. |3 was replaced by bridge. Patient aged 17.

buccal bow. Clasping problems also arise, as much space is taken up with bows in the buccal sulcus.

Self-supporting springs are best made of 0·7-mm. wire as this is strong enough to withstand the normal pressures of tongue, lips, and cheeks without further guiding or guarding and resilient enough to give a useful range of action. Springs of this type are usually made of 0·7-mm. wire and have one large coil, either near the point of attachment or between the arms if two arms are used.

The palatal movement of upper and lower canines and premolars is easily performed with

This is perfectly true, but the extra length of wire does make the spring more flexible and increases the range of action of the free end. With springs like this, which are made of comparatively thick wire, it is important to remember that their range of action is short. It is, therefore, necessary not to activate the springs too strongly in order to achieve a long range of action. These springs must be used with small adjustments made at short intervals of about two to three weeks. The disadvantage of such a short range of action is made up for by the simplicity of the spring and the positive manner of its action. *Fig.* 111 shows the correction of the bucco-lingual relation of teeth in the buccal segments.

For moving molars lingually the spring shown in *Fig.* 112 is more suitable because the sulcus, especially in the lower arch, is spring is small, and small and frequent adjustments must be made to it to keep the tooth moving.

A feature that is common to all these springs is that the spring wire comes over one

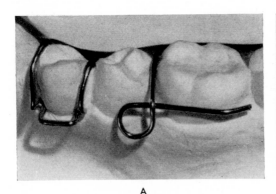
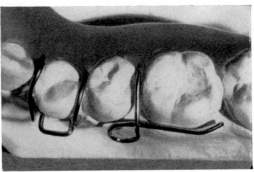

| A | B |

Fig. 112.—**A,** Self-supporting spring for lingual movement of lower molar; **B,** The plate must be left thick enough to allow trimming to let $\overline{6}$ move lingually. N.B.: $\overline{7}$ is part of the anchorage system.

shallow in the molar region and the coil of this spring is designed so as not to encroach too much on the sulcus. It is true that the end of this spring moves over a longer distance than the part near the coil, but this discrepancy can be adjusted if necessary as the tooth moves. Here again the range of action of the of the embrasures formed by the tooth that is actually being moved. This wire can easily be arranged not to interfere with the movement of the tooth or with the occlusion. The plate must be made sufficiently thick to allow for trimming away so that the tooth can move lingually.

CHAPTER VIII

MESIODISTAL MOVEMENT OF TEETH

IN performing mesiodistal movement of teeth with removable appliances, the all-important consideration is the position of the tooth apices.

The mesiodistal movement of teeth with removable appliances is not difficult to carry out as far as the crowns are concerned, but because the movement produced is a tipping one the difficulty may arise that while the crown of the tooth being moved may come to rest in the required position the resulting inclination of the root axis may be undesirable.

to consider carefully their axial inclination before any movement is attempted.

Mesiodistal tooth movement can be performed with the straightforward cantilever and self-supporting springs that have already been described. It is only necessary to place them so that their free ends move in the appropriate planes.

MESIODISTAL MOVEMENT OF UPPER INCISORS AND CANINES

The plain cantilever spring of 0·5-mm. wire is very satisfactory for this purpose, the addition of a single coil gives the spring a range of

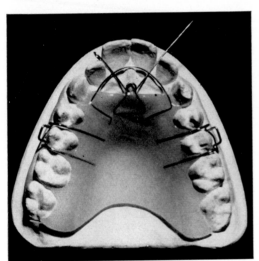

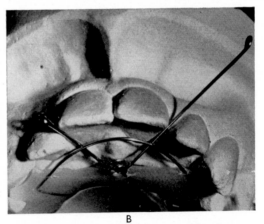

A   B

Fig. 113.—**A**, Distal movement of incisors and canines. The baseplate is made of clear material to show embedding of tags and wires. Note that the baseplate is cut back to facilitate adjustment of the spring. **B**, The two coils may if necessary be made to overlie each other. It so happens that the points of attachment of these springs coincide. Note that the guide wire holds the spring close to the gum.

The effect is seen to occur naturally in cases in which teeth have been lost prematurely and the crowns of the adjoining teeth have tipped together, the apices remaining approximately in their original positions. It is true that to some extent the root of a tooth that has been tipped mesially or distally will tend to follow the crown, but the strength of this tendency cannot be predicted with any certainty. It is important, therefore, when moving teeth mesially or distally with removable appliances,

action that will permit it to act for periods of up to a month. It is important when constructing an appliance to see that the fixed end of the spring is so placed that the moving end travels along the line of the arch as far as possible and to see that the point of application of the spring is truly on the mesial or distal surface of the tooth.

Fig. 113 **A** shows an appliance which would be used to move the upper lateral incisors distally. It so happens that in order to make

75

the springs of a suitable length and to make the points of attachment appropriate, the coils of these springs overlap one another (*Fig.* 113 B). If the points of attachment are moved outward in a radial direction to avoid the overlapping of the coils, which may be thought to

to cut back the baseplate so that adequate space is left to make adjustments to the springs. If only one spring is to be provided, the spring and guard can be made from one piece of wire, as in *Fig.* 119, and the baseplate should be similarly cut back.

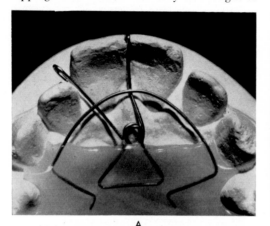

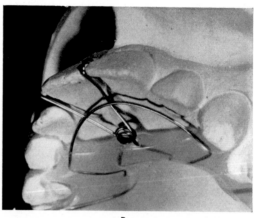

A   B

Fig. 114.—**A**, One of the springs in *Fig.* 113 has been brought over to work on the central incisor. In this way two or three teeth may be moved successively with one spring. **B**, There being no space between 1|1 the wire must be brought closely over the contact point between them and activated in an upward direction. The spring will then work its way up on to the mesial surface of the tooth. Note how the end of the wire is turned over to present a smooth end to the lip.

be technically simpler, it will be found that the springs are too short and have a limited range of action.

The springs are left long and projecting until the plate has been processed; the projecting wire is embedded in plaster in the flask and stabilizes the spring during the packing operation. When the plate is fitted the springs are finished by making a large loop which projects well into the sulcus. Such a loop does not irritate the lip unless it is allowed to project excessively. On the other hand, a cut end of wire, if left projecting ever so slightly into the sulcus, will immediately produce a spot of ulceration on the lip or cheek. The method of finishing springs by turning the end over is universal for springs of a radial type projecting into the sulcus.

As is usual with springs of this calibre and design, a guard is provided which protects and guides the spring throughout its range of action. In this appliance where two springs are formed from one piece of wire the guard can be made as a separate wire. It is important

Fig. 114 A shows how a spring can be used on more than one tooth as occasion demands. In this instance the spring used on the left upper lateral incisor has been transferred to the central incisor. It could alternatively be used on the canine if that tooth is accessible from the palatal side. The point of this arrangement is that where a number of front teeth are to be retracted one at a time, a single appliance can be used to perform these several successive movements. It is not feasible to move two incisors distally, for instance, by pushing on the first and expecting both to move distally keeping in good alinement.

If the incisors are closely in contact and a spring cannot be made to run between them, it is then necessary to run the spring over the contact point between the teeth very closely indeed so that it is not bitten on by the opposing teeth (*Fig.* 114 B), and then to activate the spring gently in an upward direction so that by pressing on the contact point it moves the teeth apart and comes to lie between them.

76

It is then possible to apply the spring to the side of the tooth and activate it laterally to produce the required distal movement.

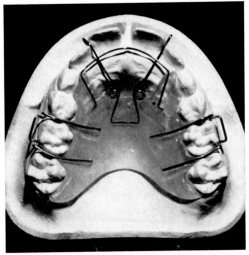

Fig. 115.—Mesial movement of teeth. The springs operate from approximately the same points, but the coils have been put on the other side. With fine springs like these it is better to cause the spring to act by opening its coil. The spring is compressed by tightening the coil.

of further winding up the coil. Practical experience shows that fine springs, that is to say of gauge 0·5 mm. and smaller, operate better if they are compressed against the coil in this way rather than in the opposite direction. Thicker springs, i.e., 0·6 mm. or larger, are found to operate equally well in both directions.

Canines may be retracted, as already mentioned, from the palatal aspect provided that they are accessible to a palatal spring. This means that the canine needs to be almost fully erupted and in normal alinement with the lateral incisor. In many cases the canine erupts high up in the sulcus and overlaps the lateral incisor so that the mesial contact point cannot be conveniently reached from the palatal aspect. In such cases the canine is more easily moved by means of a self-supporting spring in the sulcus, made of 0·7-mm. wire (*Fig.* 116 A). The free end of the spring should be turned in at right angles and applied accurately to the mesial surface of the tooth. If the canine is in close contact with the distal surface of the lateral incisor the end of the wire should be flattened anteroposteriorly by grinding so

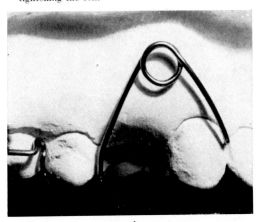

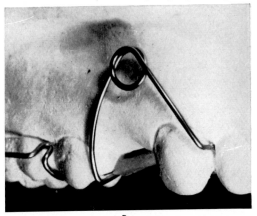

A   B

Fig. 116.—A, The buccal canine retractor. Note that the front leg of the spring will act in a backward and not a downward direction. B, The operating end of the retractor is flattened and bears accurately on or above the mesial contact point.

Fig. 115 shows an appliance designed for the mesial movement of upper central incisors. It will be noticed that the coil of the spring has been turned round so that after the spring has been activated the movement of compressing the spring to insert the appliance has the effect

that it can be inserted between the teeth and applied precisely to the mesial surface of the canine (*Fig.* 116 B). It should be noticed that the coil is disposed midway between the two arms of the spring in a mesiodistal direction and it should be arranged that this is so or so that the coil is well forward. If the coil is placed too far back, the movement of the free end of the spring becomes a downward rather than a backward one. If the canine is placed high other tooth in the arch is incorporated in the anchorage segment, it is quite possible to retract the canines without disturbing the anchorage teeth.

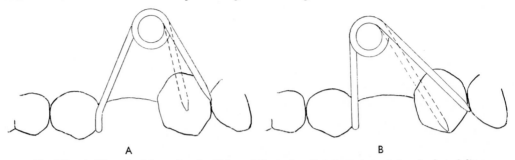

Fig. 117.—**A**, The coil of the spring should be well forward so that the spring acts in a backward direction. **B**, If the coil is too far back and the end is applied to the mesial slope of the tooth the spring will slip ineffectually down the tooth and exert no distal pressure.

up in the sulcus the second arm of the spring will have to be short and it will be of greater importance than ever to see that the coil of the spring is not too far back. A spring of this kind is effective only if it is borne in mind that it has a limited range of action, usually about one-third of the mesiodistal diameter of the tooth and provided the active end of the spring is applied precisely to the tooth at or above the mesial contact point. If the spring is applied below the contact point it is very liable to slip down the sloping mesial surface of the cusp and become ineffective (*Fig.* 117 **A**, **B**). Furthermore, the practice of hooking the spring around the mesial surface of the canine in a vague and hopeful manner is equally ineffective in most instances as a spring formed in this way is very likely to slip down on to the mesial slope of the tooth. The spring *must* be applied precisely to the tooth and given activations of not more than 2–2·5 mm. Frequent inspections will be required, that is at intervals of about three weeks, but so efficacious is this spring that the inconvenience of frequent visits is fully justified.

In retracting upper canines anchorage is a major consideration because of the large size of the roots of these teeth and of the consequent tendency of the anchorage to move rather than the canines. If the baseplate is properly designed, however (*Fig.* 118), so that every

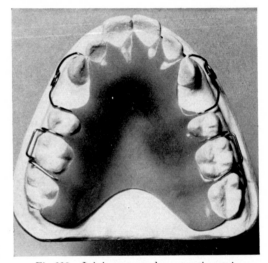

Fig. 118.—It is important when retracting canines to have adequate anchorage, otherwise the teeth in the buccal segments tend to come forward.

The buccal canine retractor just described may also be used for mesial movement of canines as it will operate equally well in either direction.

THE MESIODISTAL MOVEMENT OF UPPER PREMOLARS AND MOLARS

The simple straight cantilever spring can be used exclusively for mesiodistal movement of premolars and molars. The usual pattern of spring embodies a coil and a guard all made from the same piece of wire (*Fig.* 119). For retraction of premolars a spring of 0·5-mm. wire is most suitable, providing a very useful

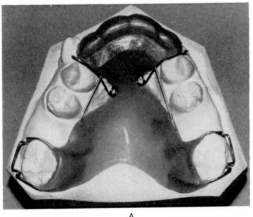

Fig. 119.—Retraction of an upper first premolar. This appliance can be fitted before the second premolar is removed and uncontrolled forward drift of teeth is thereby avoided.

and to have the free end of the arm moving as directly as possible along the line of the arch. It is also necessary to make sure that the spring impinges on the mesial surface of the tooth.

The end of the spring which projects into the buccal sulcus should be turned into a

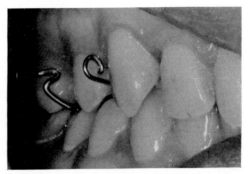

Fig. 120.—The projecting end of the premolar retractor is turned in a large loop which does not irritate the lip.

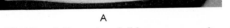
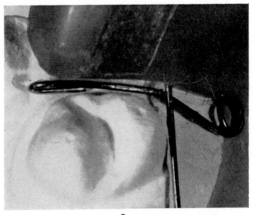

A   B

Fig. 121.—**A**, Retraction of all four upper premolars. Note that every other available tooth has been used for anchorage. The incisors are covered by the plate, so providing "stationary anchorage". **B**, Note the way in which the premolar retractor has been introduced between the lateral incisor and the premolar while keeping clear of the baseplate. Accurate waxing up and careful flasking avoid tedious trimming of acrylic from around the springs and frequent and unnecessary damage to wires which can result from the use of burs and saws.

range of action combined with a suitable pressure. The usual degree of activation for a spring of this kind is up to the full mesiodistal diameter of the premolar. It is important when laying out a spring of this kind to consider with some care its point of attachment

large loop in order to avoid injury to the inner surface of the lip (*Fig.* 120).

In certain instances when it is not possible to select the point of attachment of the spring precisely, it may be necessary to crank the spring to bring the moving end to lie squarely against the mesial surface of the tooth (*Fig.* 121).

The appliance shown in *Fig.* 119 is designed to be finished and fitted before the extraction of the right upper second premolar is carried out. Once the extraction is done, the spring can then be activated and movement of the first premolar takes place. If construction of the appliance is left until the extraction is done

the pressure used to move the premolars. Furthermore the mere question of retention of such an appliance in the arch is a difficult one to answer.

In the case under discussion the second molars are erupted sufficiently to clasp; in the anterior region the appliance is firmly supported by making the baseplate in the form of a Sved bite-plate. In this way several

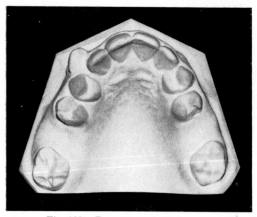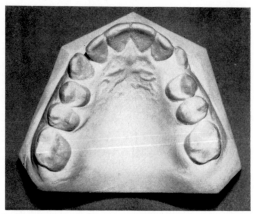

Fig. 122.—Retraction of all four premolars. Before and after. Canine space which was completely lost has been completely regained. No proclination of incisors occurred.

and delay should occur in the fitting of the appliance, movement of teeth may take place, making it impossible to get the appliance into position.

It may be necessary to free the occlusion of the teeth in the buccal segments in order to allow distal movement of premolars. This, if necessary, would be done by means of a bite plane which could be situated in the incisor or the molar region.

If both the first and the second premolars have to be moved distally it is perfectly feasible to move them together, if they are in good alinement, by means of a single spring. *Fig.* 121 illustrates the distal movement of all four upper premolars by means of removable appliances, the first permanent molars having been lost. In a case like this the problem of anchorage is a major one, because only the second molars and the incisors are available for this purpose. The second molars have a strong tendency to come forward and the incisors may procline under the reaction of

purposes are served: the appliance is held rigidly and accurately in position; an anterior bite plane is provided which releases the interlock of the premolars; "stationary anchorage" is obtained by preventing the upper incisors from proclining under the influence of the reaction. In this way it is possible to retract upper premolars without at the same time producing any forward movement of anchorage and without losing space from behind (*Fig.* 122).

If the second molars are either unerupted or not erupted sufficiently to be clasped, a further difficulty arises as it is not usually wise to use a Sved plate alone as retention for a plate used to retract four premolars, or only the four incisors as anchorage for such a tooth movement. In such a case it is best to clasp the first premolars, using them and the incisors as anchorage, and to retract the second premolars. When the second premolars are back in their new position they may be clasped and used, with the incisors, as anchorage to retract the first premolars.

Distal movement of first or second molars can be performed with a finger spring operating from the palate in the same way as for premolars. It must, of course, be decided beforehand how far it is feasible to tilt a molar distally because, if its apices are forward in position, to tip the crown distally will produce

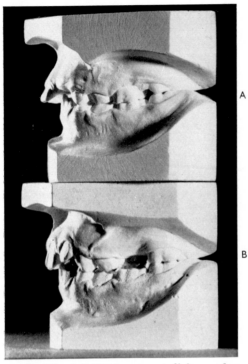

Fig. 123.—A, B, Distal movement of left upper first permanent molar, the second deciduous molar being removed. In A the upper distobuccal cusp can be seen articulating with the lower mesiobuccal cusp.

a most unnatural and unstable position for the tooth.

In *Fig.* 123 A the left upper first permanent molar has moved forward and is impacted beneath the shell of the second deciduous molar. The distobuccal cusp of the upper molar can be seen occluding with the mesiobuccal cusp of the lower. The crown of the deciduous molar was removed, the roots being completely resorbed, and by means of the appliance shown in *Fig.* 124 the molar was moved distally to its proper position (*Fig.* 123 B).

In some cases where the upper first permanent molar is impacted below the distal bulge of the second deciduous molar and cannot erupt and it is not yet time to remove the second deciduous molar, the patient being perhaps but 7 years old or thereabouts, the impacted tooth can often be freed by tying a

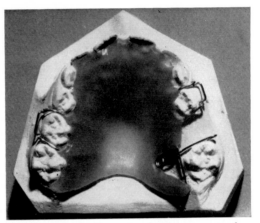

Fig. 124.—Appliance for distal movement of upper molar in *Fig.* 123.

separating wire around the contact point between the two teeth. Sometimes, however, the impaction is too severe and the separating wire cannot be put in place. In these circumstances the first permanent molar may be disimpacted by means of the following simple appliance.

The active part of the appliance is a very stiff spring of 0·9 or 1·0 mm. wire, the free end of which is flattened mesiodistally by grinding and is then carefully rounded and smoothed. The spring is arched over the gum margin and made to dip into the gingival trough in the embrasure between the first molar and second deciduous molar. (*Fig.* 125.)

When the appliance is processed and fitted, the spring is further adjusted by bending the tip down into the gingival trough, as this final adjustment cannot be properly made on the plaster cast. The spring is then activated distally a very small amount, about 0·5–1·0 mm. The spring is very stiff so that a larger adjustment would give too great a pressure. When the appliance is placed in position the spring simply slips into position by sliding up the

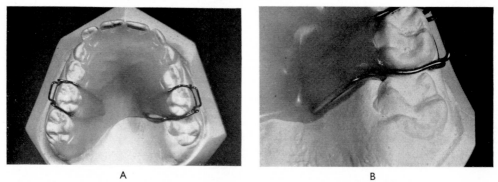

A   B

Fig. 125.—The disimpaction of a left upper first permanent molar at age 10. **A**, The general appearance of the appliance showing clasping and anchorage. **B**, Detail of the short stiff spring which clips into the gingival trough mesial to |6.

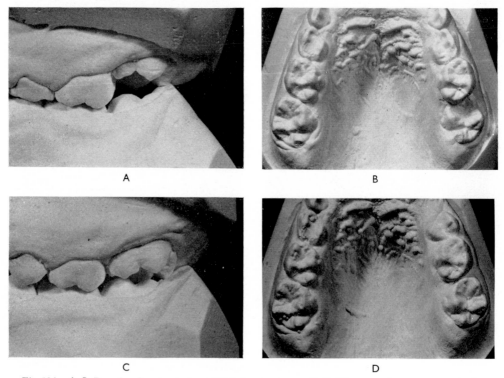

A   B

C   D

Fig. 126.—**A, B**, Buccal and occlusal views of |6 before treatment; **C, D**, The same after treatment. Active treatment time 5 months.

curving mesial surface of the first permanent molar.

Adjustments are made at intervals of 3–4 weeks depending on progress of the distal movement of the first molar. When the tooth is well disimpacted, the spring is released a little and the molar, if not already in occlusion, will then come down to the correct level. (*Fig.* 126.)

It is sometimes convenient to move a single molar distally by means of a screw. The illustrations (*Fig.* 127 **A, B**) are largely self-

82

explanatory. Anchorage is derived from the premolar or premolars mesial to the molar, the labial segment, and, to some extent, from the teeth on the other side of the arch. In the upper arch the palate will play a part in this

against anchorage, and may become mesio-distal expansion in the buccal segment concerned, with movement occurring in both groups of teeth, those in front as well as those behind the screw. This possibility must not be overlooked.

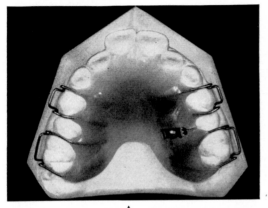
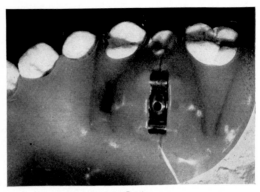

Fig. 127.—A, Distal movement of a molar by means of a screw. Note the adequate clasping of the appliance especially on either side of the site of opening of the screw. The clasping of the appliance and contact of the baseplate with the teeth all round the arch provides adequate anchorage. B, The cut in the baseplate comes out at the posterior edge at right angles which minimizes the possibility of breaking off small pieces of the baseplate at this situation.

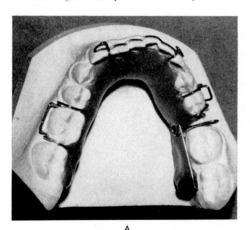
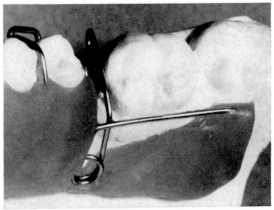

Fig. 128.—A, Distal movement of right lower second permanent molar, third molar to be extracted. Note accurately fitting labial bow for increased anchorage. B, The spring is clearly shown with a guide wire which also serves to guide the second molar. Note that the baseplate is well cut away, but for strength the spring is to be plastered in and covered with a thin layer of acrylic which makes the plate continuous in this region.

connexion. The same kind of appliance can be used in the lower arch. If the number and size of teeth on either side of the screw tend to balance evenly—if, for instance, the second molar is erupted—the movement may cease to be a simple movement of a tooth or teeth

MESIODISTAL MOVEMENT OF LOWER INCISORS AND CANINES

Movement of lower incisors in a mesial or distal direction is not conveniently performed with removable appliances and is rarely if ever done in this way. The reasons for this appear

83

to be, first, that, if lower incisor crowding is treated by extraction in the buccal segments and the canines are retracted, the incisors spread out of their own accord into the space so provided. Secondly, where extractions have been performed in the lower incisor segments and subsequent mesiodistal adjustment of position is required, this movement so often

of the arm that impinges on the tooth must be bent horizontally at right angles to the first part of the spring. A guard and guide wire is employed as for all the other springs of this type. A wide segment of the plate should be left open to facilitate adjustment of the spring, but as the baseplate is left very narrow at the lower edge (*Fig.* 128 **B**), it is best to

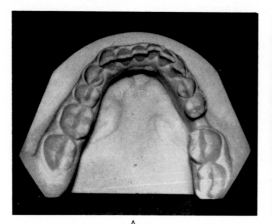
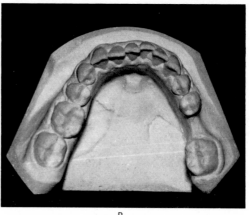

A

B

Fig. 129.—**A, B,** Distal movement of right lower second permanent molar. The first molar space has been almost completely regained and is to be bridged. No forward movement of the anterior segment occurred.

takes the form of root movement that fixed appliances must necessarily be used.

Mesial and distal movement of lower canines is, however, very often required and can be performed with a removable appliance of the same type as is used to retract upper canines from the buccal aspect. The lower labial sulcus is shallow in the canine region so that a short spring must be made, and from this it follows that only a short range of action is available. If this is kept in mind, and small adjustments made between visits, lower canines can be moved mesially and distally without difficulty.

MESIODISTAL MOVEMENT OF LOWER MOLARS AND PREMOLARS

These teeth may be moved mesially and distally in the same way as upper molars and premolars, but it must be remembered that they have an even stronger tendency to tilt. The springs are formed in exactly the same way as for upper teeth, but as the loop and first part of the arm of the spring must be placed vertically in the lingual sulcus, the part

plaster in the spring and cover it with a thin layer of wax and subsequently acrylic baseplate. This is purely to strengthen the plate in this position, the function of guiding the spring being subserved by the guide wire placed already for that purpose. *Fig.* 129 shows the effect of moving a right lower second permanent molar distally. The third molar was removed as food packing was occurring between it and the second molar. When the second molar had been moved distally, the first molar was replaced by a bridge.

It was found in this case that the reaction from the pressure required to move the second molar was producing further imbrication of the lower incisors. This was prevented and the anchorage segment stabilized as a whole by fitting a very accurate labial bow which locked the whole incisor segment from canine to canine. This bow was fitted as near as possible to the incisal edges of the teeth and reduced or prevented any tendency of the incisors to procline. This increased resistance to proclination increased the anchorage to a very great extent.

84

CHAPTER IX

EXPANSION

THE value of expansion as a treatment measure is a subject into which it is not proposed to enter here. The purpose of this chapter is to discuss the various means for producing this movement with removable appliances when the decision to expand has been made.

The term "expansion" is usually taken to mean an increase in the width of the dental arch as a whole. As the movement involved is a buccal movement of the teeth in the buccal segments, it follows that a labial movement of the incisor and canine teeth is an expansion in an anteroposterior direction. The tooth movements in these two instances differ slightly in so far as lateral expansion involves movement of the buccal segments equal distances in opposite directions; the force used and the reaction from it cause equal and opposite tooth movements; while when antero-posterior expansion is carried out the force used produces proclination of the incisors and the reaction to it will produce, or tend to produce, a distal movement of the teeth in the buccal segments. The relative amounts of movement in the labial and the buccal segments will depend on the number of teeth included in each segment. If, for instance, the whole of each buccal segment is included in the distal section of the appliance, it is unlikely that much or any distal movement of these segments will occur when even all four incisors are being moved labially.

The parts played by bucco- and labio-lingual movement and mesiodistal movement in expansion procedures should always be clearly appreciated.

The "expansion" required to regain space in the buccal segments lost as a consequence of premature removal of deciduous teeth is a complex procedure involving mesial and distal movement of the teeth in the buccal segments and labial inclination of the labial segment.

Anchorage problems do not as a rule arise, as expansion implies that simultaneous equal and opposite movements are being carried out. The force employed and its reaction are therefore both being made to do useful work.

LATERAL EXPANSION OF THE UPPER ARCH

Expansion of the upper arch can be carried out by means of a simple baseplate with a screw placed so as to act in a transverse

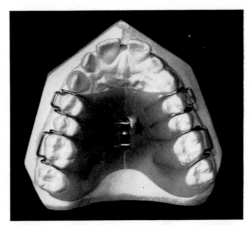

Fig. 130.—The upper screw expansion appliance, generally known as the "Badcock plate". An equal amount of expansion is produced anteriorly and posteriorly. The arrow indicates the direction in which the screw should be turned.

direction (*Fig.* 130). The screw should be placed midway between the most anterior point and the most posterior point on either side at which pressure is to be exerted. This is necessary so that as far as possible leverage on the screw is avoided. Leverage leads to the imposition of bending forces on the screw and in consequence the risk of a fracture.

If different degrees of expansion are required at the front and at the back of the buccal segments an expansion-arch type of appliance should be used.

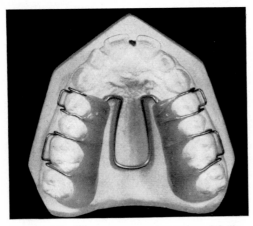

Fig. 131.—The upper expansion arch or "Coffin spring". The small registration pits can be seen anteriorly and posteriorly. The archwire is 1·25 mm. thick.

An appliance of this kind was described by Walter H. Coffin in 1881, and the arch or spring which produces the force or pressure is to-day commonly known as the Coffin spring.

large enough to make contact with all the teeth to be moved and to contain the tags of the clasps and the ends of the archwire (*Fig.* 131).

The archwire is of 1·25-mm. thickness and is formed with a generous loop in the centre; it stands 1·0 mm. away from the soft tissue of the palate. The archwire is usually made first and the tags of the clasps looped over it before waxing up the baseplate. Four small pits should be drilled with a very fine rosehead bur at each extremity of the baseplate, and these are used as registration points for recording, by means of dividers, the amount of expansion or activity given to the appliance before it is inserted.

The amount of activation given to such an appliance before insertion will depend on the length and thickness of the archwire and on the number of teeth being moved. Experience shows, however, that a range of activity of 2·0–4·0 mm. (1·0–2·0 mm. each side) is usually sufficient at a time, and further degrees of expansion are effected by subsequent adjustments.

Before any adjustment is made to an appliance of this kind the width between the registration point anteriorly and pos-

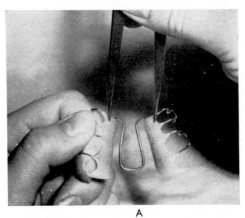
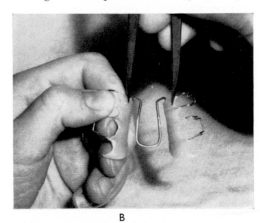

A   B

Fig. 132.—Registration of the expansion imparted to the upper expansion arch. A, Before activation; B, After activation.

Originally the baseplate was made in one piece and cut down the midline with a fine saw after vulcanizing. Present-day practice is to make the baseplate in two small segments,

teriorly should be measured with dividers and recorded. The amount of expansion given to the appliance will then be known (*Fig.* 132).

Adjustment of the appliance is effected by grasping the centre of the arch with Adams universal pliers and squeezing firmly, when the anterior end of the appliance will expand squeezing it will not do, as the arch does not run horizontally in this section and making the adjustment in this way will have the effect of tipping the distal end of the appliance

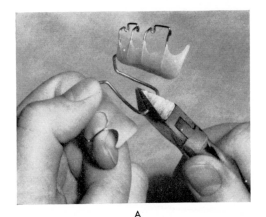

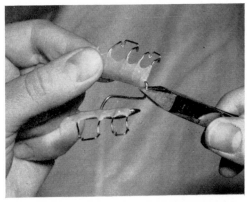

A

B

Fig. 133.—Adjustment of the upper expansion arch: A, Slight straightening of the archwire at the spot grasped in the pliers produces an expansion at the anterior end of the appliance. B, Adjustment for expansion at the posterior end is effected for each side separately. The archwire is held firmly at the spot shown and the posterior end of the appliance moved laterally in a horizontal plane. The other side is adjusted similarly.

(Fig. 134 A). Expansion of the posterior ends is effected by opening the appliance about the anterior ends of the arch. It is necessary to make this adjustment by grasping a straight section of away from the palate as well as laterally. If both ends of the appliance are adjusted in this way and hence tipped, the effect will be to tip the loop of the arch into

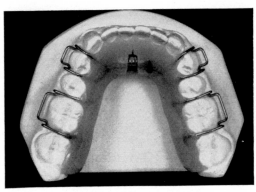

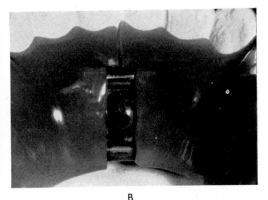

A

B

Fig. 134.—A, The lower screw expansion appliance or lower Badcock plate. B, The screw for this appliance. There is considerable bending stress imposed on the screw in this appliance by the long arms extending distally to the molar region.

the arch in the pliers and bending the distal end of the appliance laterally (Fig. 133 B). Making the adjustment by grasping a bend in the arch at the front with the pliers and the palate. Making an adjustment at the anterior ends of the appliance by squeezing only is very likely to introduce warpage and distortion.

LATERAL EXPANSION OF THE LOWER ARCH

Lateral expansion of the lower arch can be effected with a screw type of appliance with the screw placed in the middle line behind the

appliance very efficient but an easily controlled difference in expansion can be effected anteriorly or posteriorly (*Fig.* 135).

As with the upper arch expansion appliance, the baseplate is only large enough to contain

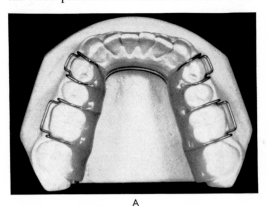

A

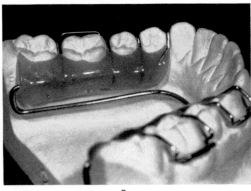

B

Fig. 135.—**A,** The lower expansion arch or Coffin spring. **B,** The disposition of the arch in the premolar and molar region.

incisors (*Fig.* 134). With this arrangement, however, leverage on the screw is very great and any bending of the screw will result in lack of expansion at the distal parts of the arch.

the ends of the arch and the tags of the clasps. The arch is again 1·25 mm. thick and registration pits are made at the ends of the baseplate. Adjustment of the appliance is effected in much the same way as the upper type of

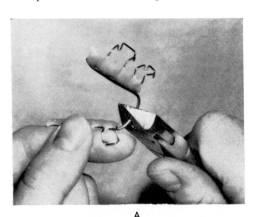

A

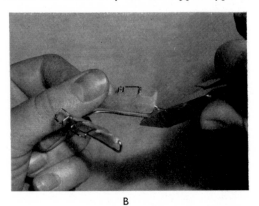

B

Fig. 136.—Adjustment of the lower expansion arch. **A,** For adjustment posteriorly the middle section of the arch is straightened slightly by grasping firmly with Adams universal pliers. **B,** The anterior ends are adjusted by grasping each posterior end firmly as shown and adjusting the anterior end in a horizontal direction. Registration of expansion is carried out as shown in *Fig.* 133.

The screw is in fact at a great disadvantage in trying to operate through such a long arm at either side.

A better arrangement is to use the expansion-arch type of appliance. Not only is this

appliance. The posterior ends of the appliance are expanded by grasping the curved horizontal middle section of the arch with Adams universal pliers (*Fig.* 136 A). Adjustment of the anterior ends is made for each side separately while gripping the distal ends of the arch firmly by a section that cannot be distorted by pressure of the pliers (*Fig.* 136 B). The range of activity should be of the order of 2·0–4·0 mm. at a time, further expansion being effected by subsequent adjustment.

ANTEROPOSTERIOR EXPANSION

As mentioned earlier, the proclination of all the incisors amounts to an expansion in an anteroposterior direction (*see* pp. 63 – 66) although in such a procedure movement is usually limited to the incisors and the reaction is dissipated over the teeth in the buccal segments. There are, however, one or two special cases of anteroposterior expansion that must be mentioned.

The Upper Arch.—Where it is desired to produce anteroposterior expansion involving some labial movement of the incisor teeth and distal movement of the buccal segments, this can be effected by means of an appliance split in three directions and employing two screws. This is sometimes known as the Y appliance (*Fig.* 137). If the screws are operated simultaneously the buccal segments are moved distally and slightly laterally and

be anticipated when the effects of such an expansion are being forecast. The use of a labial bow fitting well towards the incisal

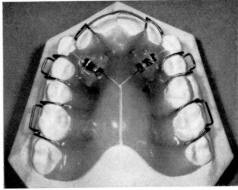

Fig. 137.—The Y appliance. Useful for opening spaces required for upper canines. The resistance of the buccal segments to movement greatly outweighs that of the incisor segments. This must be foreseen. The resistance of the upper incisor segment may be increased by fitting a labial bow near the incisal edges as shown.

edges of the teeth will, however, reduce the tendency to proclination and cause a greater effect on the teeth in the buccal segments. It will also be appreciated that the slight lateral expansion of the buccal segments

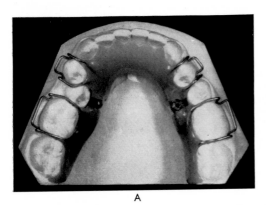

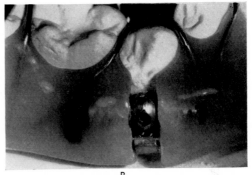

A   B

Fig. 138.—Opening spaces for lower premolars. A, Note the firm clasping of the appliance at either side of the site of expansion. If there appears to be a risk of proclining the incisors excessively, a labial bow may be used, fitted near to the incisal edges of the teeth. B, If the lingual sulcus is shallow, one guide rod may be cut off the screw. The remaining guide rod and the screw itself are usually strong enough for this particular expansion as there is little or no bending stress on the screw.

the labial segment is moved labially. The labial segment is of course outweighed by at least two to one and will tend to move rather more than the buccal segments, and this must

will facilitate their distal movement, as the teeth will be kept on the divergent alveolar ridges as they move in a distal direction.

The Lower Arch.—As already mentioned, proclination of the lower incisors is in fact an anteroposterior expansion. The opening up of space for premolars that are impacted as a result of the premature loss of deciduous

This last movement must be anticipated and allowed for as it may subsequently appear that the space gained in the buccal segments is at the expense of the incisor teeth if they do not remain in their proclined position.

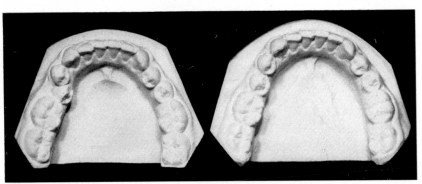

Fig. 139.—Space has been opened up for 5|5.

molars is often also referred to as expansion, although in fact the movements involved are mesially and distally in the buccal segments.

Space opening in the buccal segments can be effected by means of screws. A baseplate with a screw at the site of a collapse will produce a mesial movement of the teeth in front of the site and distal movement of the teeth behind (*Fig.* 138 A). In the labial segment a proclination will be produced.

If the lingual sulcus is shallow, a compact screw must be used, and the depth of the baseplate kept to the minimum (*Fig.* 138 B).

The appliance must be firmly clasped on either side of the site of expansion so that loss of fit as the appliance expands is avoided. The effect of opening up space in the lower arch for impacted premolars can be seen in *Fig.* 139.

A valuable paper in the treatment of collapse in the lower arch has been published by Leech (1951).

CHAPTER X

INTERMAXILLARY AND EXTRA-ORAL TRACTION

THE use of intermaxillary and extra-oral traction with removable appliances is not a new idea. Intermaxillary traction was used with removable appliances over half a century ago (Jackson, 1906) and more recently with appliances clasped with arrowhead clasps. The

claspable teeth are not present in the arch concerned, use may be made of the accessory arrowhead clasp to increase retention of the appliance. It is not so much that the appliance requires to be fiercely clasped to the teeth but that it needs to be positively supported at each corner, so that levering and tipping effects are resisted.

THE LOWER TRACTION APPLIANCE

The standard lower traction appliance is clasped on the first premolars and first permanent molars (*Fig.* 140). This ensures that the

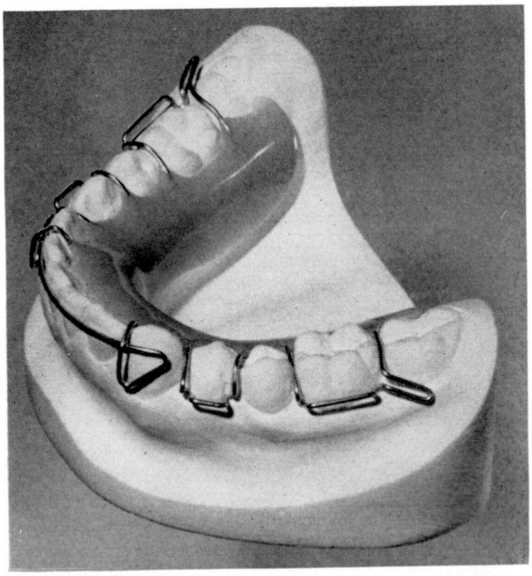

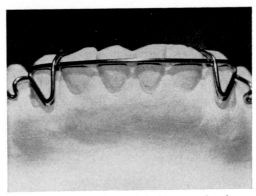

Fig. 140.—The lower traction plate. The standard traction hook is here in use. Note that the labial bow fits all teeth very accurately.

Fig. 141.—The labial bow on the lower traction plate is placed as near the incisal edges as possible.

introduction of the Adams clasp has greatly simplified the design and construction of traction appliances and made possible the use of extra-oral traction and free sliding labial arches on removable appliances.

The general design of traction plates does not differ greatly from that of ordinary upper or lower removable appliances. It will be realized that firm retention for the appliances will be necessary so that four clasps on each plate are normally required. Where four

plate will not move or lift up under the tension of the elastic traction. In some instances this ideal retention is not available because the first premolar has not erupted. It is then necessary to adopt the expedient of putting an auxiliary arrowhead clasp on a second deciduous molar. The lower traction hook on the first permanent molar may be of the standard type, or if necessary one of the special variations (Chapter VI) depending on the depth of the buccal sulcus in the molar region.

91

An indispensable feature of the lower traction plate is the labial bow. This bow is not a retention device, but serves the important purpose of preventing proclination of the lower incisors. The bow must lie accurately against the labial surfaces of the incisors

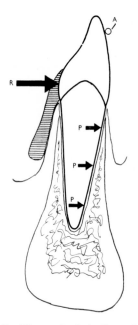

Fig. 142.—The mechanical effect of the labial bow in the lower traction plate. The reaction **R** transmitted through the baseplate tends to procline the lower incisors. The labial arch **A** prevents proclination and converts the pressure on the lower incisors into pressure P, P, P, distributed evenly over the labial alveolar bone. An element of "stationary anchorage" is thereby created.

and canines nearly at their incisal edges (*Fig.* 141). These teeth are thus prevented from inclining forward under the pressure exerted on them from behind and so become very much more resistant to movement than if they are simply permitted to tilt forward. An element of 'stationary anchorage' is therefore obtained (*Fig.* 142). This bow also locks the six front teeth into a rigid block against the baseplate and so prevents mesiodistal movement which would result in rotations and imbrications. As a result of these arrangements the lower traction plate creates out of the lower dental arch an exceedingly firm rigid

92

base from which to exert traction on the upper dentition.

The arrangement of the lower labial bow should be carefully noted. As the embrasures between the canines and the first premolars are already occupied by the wire of the premolar clasp, the tags of the bow are brought lingually between the canines and the lateral incisors. The wire used for the bow should be 0·6 mm. thick and will not interfere with the occlusion.

Both theoretically and in practice a plate of this kind when properly constructed will give more reliable anchorage from the lower arch, with less likelihood of upsetting the alinement of the front teeth, than many of the conventional appliances of the labiolingual type, and there are the additional advantages of ease and speed of construction and all the convenience of a removable appliance where cleanliness and the health of the soft and hard tissues are concerned.

UPPER TRACTION APPLIANCES

Upper traction appliances vary, depending on the kind of tooth movement required, but all consist essentially of a baseplate clasped

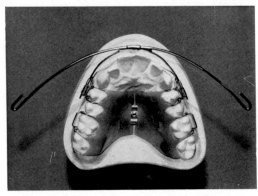

Fig. 143.—Upper traction plate for distal movement of buccal segments. If only intermaxillary traction is being used, the tubes on the premolar clasps and the extra-oral arch are unnecessary. Note the expansion screw. This is *not* necessarily for active expansion of the upper arch. Note Trevor Johnson friction-fit stops which hold the labial bow forward and free of the incisors.

to the first premolars and first molars and provided with a means of expanding the baseplate in a lateral direction. This expansion mechanism is not provided, however, for the purpose of actively expanding the arch laterally, but is for the purpose of permitting expansion of the plate following upon the distal movement of the upper buccal segments. This distal movement is usually accompanied by an expansion, because the teeth in moving distally move on to a wider part of the arch. The expansion mechanism may be either the conventional screw or the Coffin type of expansion arch.

The standard type of traction plate is clasped to the first premolars and first molars, and hooks are incorporated in the first premolar clasps. When used in this form this plate is designed to produce distal movement of the buccal segments only (*Fig.* 143). By dividing the operation of moving the upper arch distally into two stages, moving the buccal segments distally first, then retracting the upper

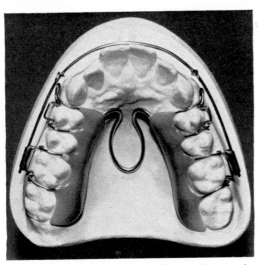

Fig. 144.—Upper traction plate for retroclination of upper incisors and canines. The free-sliding arch is of 1·0-mm. wire. Note Coffin type of expansion arch as an alternative to the screw in *Fig.* 143.

incisors and canines separately, the strain on the anchorage of the lower arch can be reduced. Lighter elastic tensions can be used to produce movement of the two parts of the upper arch than would be required if the upper arch were to be moved as a whole.

If of course it is desired to bring the lower buccal segments forward, as is required for

instance in cases where spacing occurs between the buccal segments and the canines, the lower plate is constructed with a lingual arch standing well clear of the gingival tissues behind the lower incisors and canines, and no labial arch. The whole plate can then come

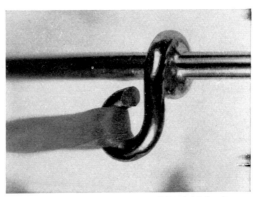

Fig. 145.—Stop hooks on free sliding labial arch on appliance in *Fig.* 144. Hooks of 0·7-mm. soft wire soldered on. Elastic in position.

forward slightly under the influence of the intermaxillary traction. It may be necessary to fit a Coffin type of lingual arch to permit contraction of the appliance a little as the buccal segments come forward, but this is not usually necessary.

When the upper buccal segments have been retracted and it is desired to retract the incisors and canines, a free-sliding labial arch may be added to the upper appliance running in tubes soldered to the molar clasps (*Fig.* 144). These tubes may be placed on the clasps from the outset in anticipation of the second phase of treatment or they may easily be added later when required.

It is necessary to make the free-sliding arch of a fairly substantial wire, 1·0 mm. or 0·9 mm. thick at least, and to match the archwire carefully with the tubing in order to ensure that the arch runs freely in the buccal tubes.

The traction hook on the buccal arch, *Fig.* 145, is also designed to serve the purpose of providing a firm and indestructible stop for extra-oral traction and is therefore called the "stop hook". It is made from 0·7-mm. soft stainless steel wire turned accurately round the archwire and soldered. The free end is then turned backwards and finished off under the arch as shown.

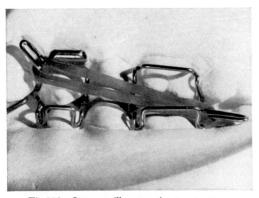

Fig. 146.—Intermaxillary traction to retract upper buccal segments. Note how elastic comes from distal aspect of lower molar to mesial aspect of upper premolar and elastic lies almost horizontally.

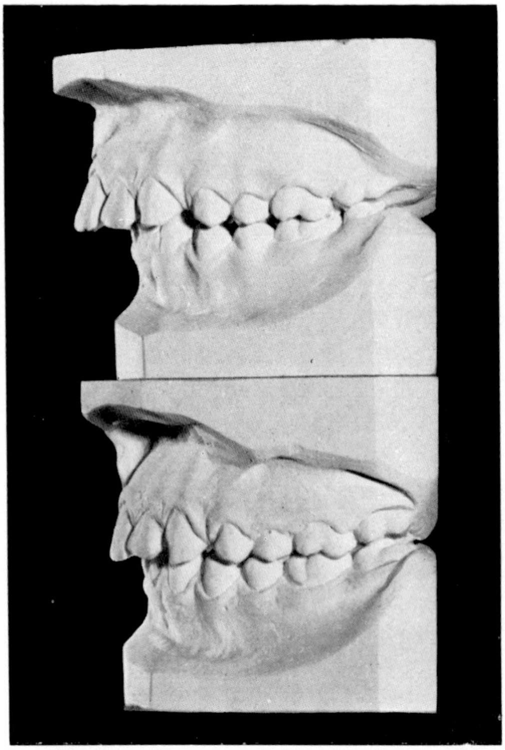

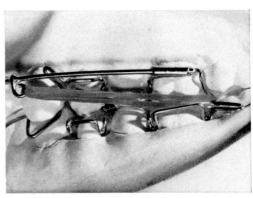

Fig. 147.—Intermaxillary traction to upper free-sliding arch to retract upper incisors. Note that traction is almost horizontal.

It will be seen that the intermaxillary traction produced by both these upper traction appliances and the standard lower traction appliance is almost horizontal when the teeth are in occlusion and there is very little vertical component (*Figs.* 146, 147).

When the distal movement of the upper arch is carried out as a two-stage operation—distal movement of the buccal segments followed by retroclination of the upper incisors and canines—it may be considered necessary to stabilize the buccal segments during the second stage of treatment in case there is any tendency to relapse. This can be done by placing coil springs on the upper free-sliding buccal arch between the stop hooks and the molar tubes.

These coil springs should be of very fine wire, 0·15 mm. thick, and lie between the distal aspect of the stop hooks and the mesial ends of the tubes. When slightly compressed the springs will exert the necessary gentle stabilizing pressure on the buccal segments. The main pressure will continue to be exerted by the arch anteriorly on the incisors. The correction of the buccal segment and incisor relation in *Fig.* 148 was carried out as a two-stage operation using intermaxillary traction alone.

EXTRA-ORAL TRACTION

The tendency for intermaxillary traction to upset the lower arch by bringing buccal

Fig. 148.—Treatment of Class II, div. 1 malocclusion with intermaxillary traction. This was done as a two-stage operation. No stabilization of buccal segments was used during the second phase of treatment.

segments forward and producing imbrication of incisors is well known. This tendency can be reduced or eliminated by careful construction

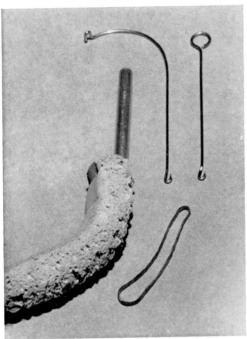

Fig. 149.—The rigid-tube cervical traction attachment. This shows exactly half of the tubular collar and two types of extra-oral arm. The sorbo rubber is sewn on while the tube, 12 in. by $\frac{1}{4}$ in. duralumin tube, is straight. The tube and rubber are then bent to fit the patient's neck, avoiding the angles of the mandible. A sufficient length at the sides must be left straight in which the wire arms (1·25 mm. thick) will run. The elastic is 2–3 in. by $\frac{1}{16}$ in.–$\frac{1}{8}$ in. wide and is pulled through with a length of 0·6-mm. wire, the inside of the tube being well dusted with french chalk.

of the lower appliance and judicious adjustment of the tension applied to the lower arch.

The use of extra-oral traction as the main moving pressure in retraction of the upper arch, with intermaxillary traction as a day-time stabilizing pressure only, practically eliminates any risk of seriously upsetting the lower dental arch.

There is a strong tendency to-day to depend less on intermaxillary traction for the correction of buccal segment relations and to use extra-oral traction to expedite treatment and reduce stress on the lower

arch. It has been found, however, that the use of day-time intermaxillary traction to stabilize advances gained on the upper arch

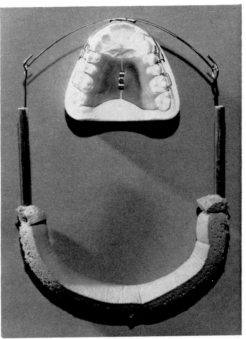

Fig.150.—Extra-oral traction for distal movement of upper buccal segments. The extra-oral wires are 1·25 mm. thick, the small labial bow 1·0 mm. thick. The tubes are soldered to the premolar clasps and the small labial bow plugs in to the tubes. The labial bow is prevented from touching the upper incisors by means of friction fit movable stops. (See also Figs. 81, 143.)

during the night is an important detail that should not be omitted.

THE EXTRA-ORAL HEADGEAR

Many different kinds of extra-oral headgear have been described in the past, but they all fall into one of two general types, the cervical type and the headcap type. The only difference in principle between the two is that with a headcap it is possible to vary the direction of pull to some extent, while the cervical traction collar as a rule sits in one position only on the patient's neck and tends to pull slightly in a downward direction. It is frequently found that the direction of pull is not critical and that, with removable appliances of the kind described, there is no tendency for the cervical traction to displace the upper appliance even

when the maximum grasp of the clasps is not exerted.

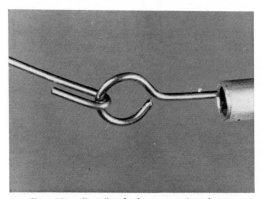

Fig. 151.—Detail of the connexion between the extra-oral wire arm and the extra-oral bow. This connexion is easily made and undone by the patient.

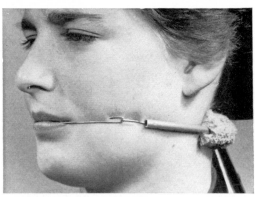

Fig. 152.—Cervical traction in position. This photograph shows an earlier form of hook connexion with the extra-oral arm. The general arrangement is otherwise the same.

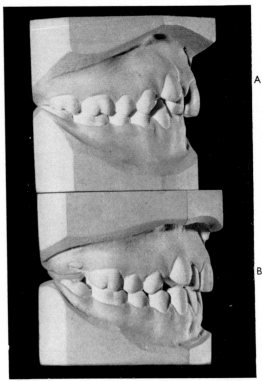

Fig. 153.—A, B, Retraction of upper buccal segments with extra-oral and intermaxillary traction. The upper second molars have been removed and the upper third molars are just appearing in B. 3|3 were brought completely into line in the arch. Patient aged 20.

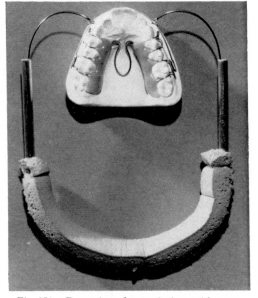

Fig. 154.—Retraction of upper incisors with extra-oral traction.

The Cervical Attachment.—A convenient form of cervical attachment is the U-shaped aluminium tube with a foam rubber strip sewn around it at the posterior part where pressure is produced on the back of the neck. This tube supports and guides the two extra-oral arms through which traction is brought to the intra-oral appliance, and contains the long elastic band from which the tension is derived (*Fig.* 149).

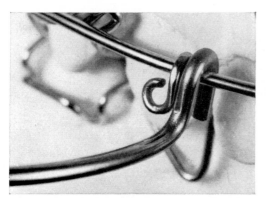

Fig. 155.—Detail showing engagement of extra-oral hook with the stop hook on the free-sliding labial bow, 1·0 mm. Stop hook 0·7-mm. soft wire.

The details of the connexion between the extra-oral attachment and the upper appliance will vary with the type of appliance in use.

For the upper appliance that is being used only to retract the upper buccal segments it is most convenient to provide an attachment which plugs into tubes soldered to the first premolar clasps (*Figs.* 143, 150). This attachment consists of a short labial arch made of 1·0-mm. wire and provided with Trevor Johnson friction fit stops (Johnson, 1952) which hold it forward and well clear of the labial surfaces of the incisors. (*See Fig.* 81.) The extra-oral bow is made from a single piece of heavy wire, 1·25 mm., which is wrapped to the smaller arch with soft fine stainless steel wire, 0·3 mm., and soldered. The ends of this bow are turned into convenient hooks.

The arms of the cervical attachment, for use in conjunction with this type of extra-oral bow, are turned into large circular loops which can be easily engaged and disengaged by the patient (*Fig.* 151). Fig. 152 shows the complete extra-oral attachment in position. An older type of connexion between the extra-oral arm and the bow of the cervical attachment is actually in use in this illustration. The extra-oral attachment can be fitted on to the plate by the patient on retiring at night and removed in the morning. Intermaxillary traction

is discontinued during the night. *Fig.* 153 A, B shows the distal movement of upper buccal segments by the methods described.

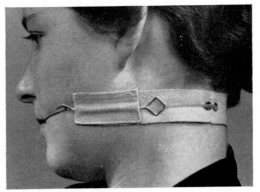

Fig. 156.—An alternative form of cervical attachment made of webbing 1 in. wide. The elastic is looped through two closely placed eyeletted holes. The extra-oral arm has a large loop on it to prevent rotation of the arm and facilitate alinement of the loop at its anterior end.

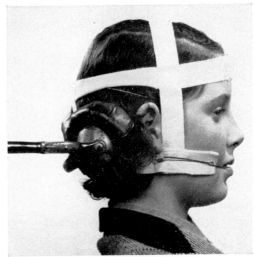

Fig. 157.—The webbing headcap. The lowermost horizontal band to which the hook and elastic are attached can be arranged at whatever height seems convenient and the direction of pull thereby controlled.

If the upper appliance is of the kind that is fitted with a free-sliding labial bow for retraction of the upper incisors, the details of the connexion with the cervical traction are slightly different. The arms which emerge from the cervical tube curve forward and

97

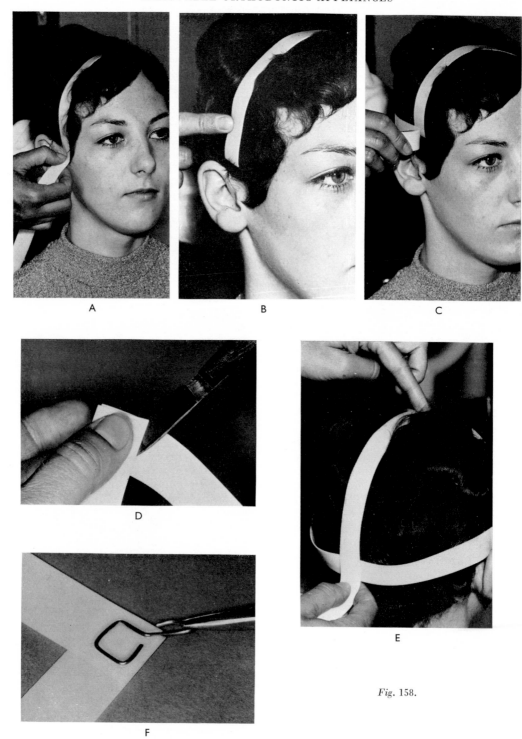

A

B

C

D

E

F

Fig. 158.

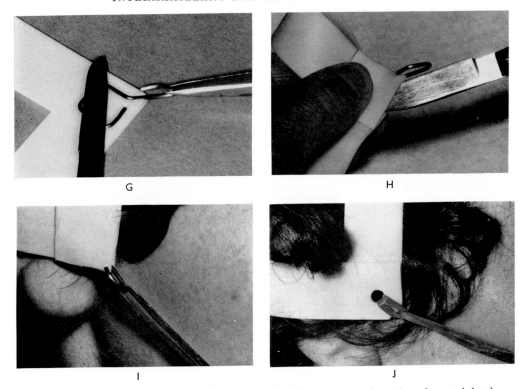

Fig. 158.—Construction of a plastic headcap. A, B, Measurement and cutting of coronal band. C, Measurement of occipital or cervical band. D, The coronal and cervical bands are joined by slipping a clean hot wax knife between the pieces of material while held lightly in contact. The joint is completed with firm finger pressure. The knife must be continually cleaned by scraping lightly as the adherent plastic material chars when the knife is re-heated and makes jointing difficult and dirty. E, The sagittal band is measured, cut, and jointed. F, G, The hooks are made of 1·25-mm. wire, heated, and pressed into the corners of the headcap. The position is adjusted to suit the angle of pull of the elastic. H, I, The hook is finally anchored with a square of material sealed over it. J, A simple way to attach extra-oral elastics to a plastic headcap is by punching a hole with a leather punch and looping the elastic through as shown. The tension can be adjusted by using different lengths and thicknesses of elastic bands.

inward and are formed into hooks which fit over the buccal arch and impinge on the front of the stop hooks (*Figs.* 154, 155). Where this appliance is in use, the patient at night removes the intermaxillary elastics and puts on the cervical traction appliance. In the morning the extra-oral traction is removed and new intermaxillary elastics put in place.

Other kinds of cervical attachment have been described and are regularly in use (McCallin, 1954). Some are made of webbing (*Fig.* 156), and others of more flexible kinds of plastic tubing. All have their advocates and are perfectly effective; it merely remains for the operator to select the one that accords best with his preferences. It will be found, however, on the whole that the curved type of extra-oral arm shown in *Fig.* 154 works best if it runs in a rigid metal tube.

The Headcap.—The webbing or net headcap has the advantage that the direction of pull may be varied in a vertical direction, and in some cases it may be thought better to have the pull coming from a higher point than would be possible with cervical traction. Headcap design varies, but the essential features are a coronal band, a horizontal band running around the brow and around the backmost part of the head, and a median sagittal band which provides a tab anteriorly

99

to help in pulling on the headcap. A second horizontal band is provided which runs around the back of the head at a level designed to give the required direction of pull. This last horizontal band is attached to the sagittal

case and the operator's own ideas, and other materials than webbing may be used in their construction.

Plastic belt material can be used successfully for headcap construction. This material

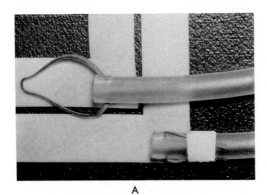

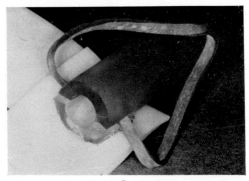

A   B

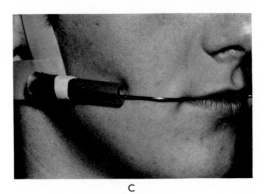

Fig. 159.—The construction of a plastic headcap with a built-in arm for the application of traction to a multiband arch or free sliding labial arch as shown in *Figs.* 144, 154, and 155. A, B, A short length of polythene tubing is sealed on to the headcap with a hot knife. The back end of the tubing is cut with a scalpel or sharp knife, and the elastic that is hooked on to the extra-oral wire arm is pulled back sufficiently and jammed in the cut end of the tubing (A, *above*, B). The end of the elastic band is turned back, taped down with adhesive plaster, and cut off (A, *below*). C, The headgear in place.

C

band posteriorly and to the ends of the coronal band laterally.

Attachment of the elastics to the headcap is effected by means of large-sized hooks of the "hook and eye" type. It is usual to use fairly short elastics, although the hooks may be placed at any point along the horizontal band of webbing to enable the operator to use any length of elastic he may wish.

The headcap is constructed by pinning or stapling it together and trying it on the patient's head, after which it is sewn permanently together and the hooks placed in position (*Fig.* 157).

The design of webbing headcaps may of course be varied according to the needs of the

is easily joined by running a clean hot wax knife between the two surfaces to be united and pressing the two parts firmly together. Heated hooks may be embedded in the material and sealed in with a hot knife.

Plastic belting material offers so many advantages in speed, adaptability, hygiene, and versatility that for many workers it is the material of choice. If thick-walled polythene tubing is also brought into use, every kind of extra-oral traction appliance can be rapidly constructed. The series of illustrations in *Fig.* 158 shows the construction of a head cap. *Figs.* 159, 160 show a number of variations that can be made, indicating the scope of the technique.

100

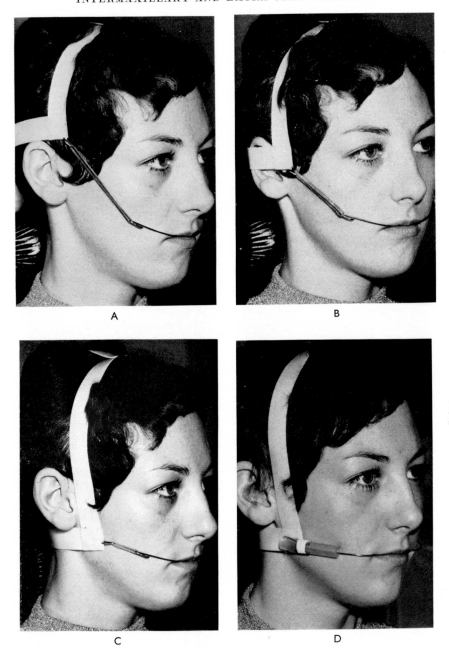

Fig. 160.—A variety of headgears can easily be made by varying the lengths of the coronal, cervical, and sagittal bands. A, High pull headgear. B, Medium pull headgear. C, Horizontal pull headgear. D, Headgear for use with fixed appliances or free sliding labial bow.

CHAPTER XI

FUNCTIONAL APPLIANCES

FUNCTIONAL JAW ORTHOPÆDICS★ is the system of orthodontic treatment which makes use of forces which act in and about the human dentition during the activities of the masticatory face. In suitable cases treatment with functional appliances offers a means of treating severe malocclusions simply, rapidly, and reliably, but it should also be borne in mind that such treatment applied to conditions for which it is not suited can be ineffectual and hence lead to waste of time and effort.

Functional jaw orthopædics embraces treatment with any of the appliances or appliance systems in which loose-fitting devices are placed between or about the teeth, so redirecting the pressures of the facial or masticatory muscles on to the teeth and their supporting structures in such ways as to produce improvements in tooth arrangements and occlusal relations.

The first and most well known, but by no means the only, systematic approach to the design and use of functional appliances was that of Andresen (1936), although it has frequently been pointed out that Robin (1902) anticipated the general shape of the appliance or 'monobloc' that is used in the Andresen System. It should always be borne in mind that whatever the name of the appliance or system that is used, the central purpose is to produce a temporary redirection of the forces that are already at play within and about the oral cavity until such time as premeditated changes in tooth arrangement and occlusal relationship have been brought about.

A slightly different approach to functional appliance treatment, which is also not lacking in precedents, is that of Fränkel (1966) in which the pressures of the tongue, lips, and cheeks are prevented from impinging upon the teeth and alveolar processes by means of a "Function Corrector" or "Function Regulator", producing in consequence changes in the growth patterns of these structures. The oral screen must properly be described as a functional appliance as also must be the bite plane, whether horizontal or inclined.

In view of the mode of action of functional appliances, it is not possible entirely to separate a discussion of their design and construction from some consideration of the nature of the irregularities and malocclusions which such appliances are used to treat and the effects which the appliances produce.

THEORETICAL PRINCIPLES

The foundation on which functional orthopædics of the jaws rests is the theory of 'functional adaptation' evolved by Roux (1895) conceived as a fundamental principle which determines the arrangement of the teeth and the form of the jaws in which the dentition is placed. Häupl, Grossmann, and Clarkson (1952) have embodied the conception of the treatment of malocclusion by functional means in their statement that: "Tissue-forming functional stimuli originate from the activity of the tongue, lip, facial, and masticatory muscles. These stimuli are transmitted to the teeth, paradontal tissue, alveolar bone, and mandibular joint through a passive, loose-fitting appliance inserted between the teeth, the result being that the transmitted stimuli induce the desired changes in the tissues affected."

The theoretical basis of the system of functional treatment suggests that the new pattern of function dictated by the appliance or activator leads to the development of a correspondingly new morphological pattern, not only of tooth arrangement and occlusion, but also of facial size and proportions. If this is indeed so, then it should be possible from the study of treated cases to show at what sites and to what degree changes in form have

---

★ *Funktionskieferorthopädie*, also known as F.K.O.

taken place within the jaws, temporomandibular joints, and dento-alveolar structures.

To-day it is widely acknowledged that dramatic and permanent improvements in occlusal relationships can be produced by functional appliances in some cases. The changes in the occlusion can be seen and estimated clinically with considerable accuracy by means of the teeth, which do not alter in size and shape, but the nature and extent of the accompanying changes in the shape of the jaws and face are much less easy to measure, especially as growth increments in these areas may have taken place at the same time as the treatment procedures were carried out.

It is believed by many advocates of functional jaw orthopædics, on the basis of clinical experience, that changes occur at the condyle of the mandible as a result of stimulation of growth at this site leading to increase in mandibular length. Korkhaus (1960), from the cephalometric examination of Class II, division 1 malocclusion treated by activators, suggested that the changes in mandibular conformation rapidly produced correction of the occlusal relationship, and hence no changes in tooth position within the jaws were necessary; not only did this make for a more stable end-result, but also there was no risk to the periodontal tissues as a result of the orthodontic treatment.

An investigation into the effects produced by functional appliances in the treatment of Class II, div. 1 malocclusion had previously been carried out by Softley (1953) with the aid of cephalometric X-ray analysis.

This author found that while, after treatment with activator appliances, considerable changes had taken place in tooth inclination, particularly upper incisor inclination and in alveolar prognathism, changes in basal prognathism, other than changes attributable to growth, could not be detected.

Moss (1962) analysed the results of activator treatment of 30 cases of Class II, div. 1 malocclusion. Using cephalometric X-ray films Moss found that in 76 per cent of cases there was a forward growth difference of the lower jaw in relation to the upper, the lower jaw growing forwards more rapidly than the upper by 1 mm. per year. Moss explained this result in terms of a releasing of inhibiting factors in the growth of the lower jaw through the use of the activator.

Björk (1963) has shown by the cephalometric X-ray study of growth and development in Class II, div. 1 cases that while the dental base relationship may remain unchanged as growth proceeds, this relationship may in some cases improve towards normality and in others deteriorate to a more severe degree of postnormality. Such growth changes as these modify to a great degree the response of cases of postnormal occlusion when treatment is carried out by activators. Favourable growth changes, taking place during treatment, accelerate the improvements in occlusal relationship brought about by functional appliances. In contrast, the absence of favourable growth changes or the deterioration in dental base relationship will delay or prevent entirely any correction of occlusal relationship by means of activator treatment.

According to Björk, "Treatment is divided into three types according to the growth trend of the sagittal jaw relationship.

"1. If the sagittal jaw relationship is postnormal but is growing towards normality, that is to say, if lower prognathism is increasing in relation to upper prognathism, then prognosis is good. In such circumstances, an activator or even a bite plate will be sufficient to produce the required result. The appliance will function by growth adaptation in that it removes distal intercuspidation and thereby makes it possible for the occlusion to develop in the normal direction in the same degree as the sagittal jaw relation. Occipital traction on the upper molars will have the same effect during growth adaptation in that the distal intercuspidation is removed. Tooth movement of other kinds is not required. In cases with normal spacing, extraction is not necessary and the treatment should be done before the end of puberal growth.

"2. Where prognathism is developing at the same rate in both jaws, the jaw relationship remains unchanged. Here it is necessary to treat the malocclusion by means of tooth movement. Fixed appliances are most useful

103

in combination with occipital traction. In such cases, occipital traction moves the teeth, and tooth movement may be easier if certain teeth are extracted in one or both jaws. Removable appliances such as the activator can be used with good prospects where there is considerable growth in alveolar height, but in these cases treatment must then be done before the end of puberal growth.

"3. If prognathism of the upper jaw is increasing in relation to the lower, treatment is difficult. Removable appliances are contra-indicated if they remove the intercuspidation which is the natural compensatory occlusal mechanism. Treatment has to be done by tooth movement with fixed appliances in combination with occipital traction and extraction in both jaws. Tooth movement has to compensate for increased deterioration in the sagittal jaw relation. For this reason, treatment may be done late, after puberal growth, and the finished treatment has to be retained with occlusal stabilization."*

It is clear that while the decision to carry out orthodontic treatment by means of functional appliances must rest to a great extent upon a multitude of clinical observations and assessments, the effects of treatment cannot be explained by anything less than the most precise measuring methods available, and much remains to be discovered about the details of the effects produced by functional appliances.

Further theoretical advantages arising from the use of functional appliances concern the reaction of the periodontal tissues to the influence of activators in pressing on the teeth. The pressure exerted by activators differs from the pressure exerted by active appliances, or appliances embodying sources of stored pressure, in that activator pressure is intermittent even while the appliance is being worn, and also this intermittent pressure is only applied for a proportion of the 24 hours, as activators are usually only worn at night. The pressure exerted by active appliances is continuous, the appliances being worn all of the 24 hours.

The effect of activators is to impose impulses or shocks to the teeth and their surrounding structures, such impulses being under the control of the masticatory muscles and hence "physiological" in character. It is thought that the physiological and momentary nature of the impulses avoids the stretching and compressing of the periodontal membrane found with the continuous pressure of active appliances. In the functional appliance system the periodontal tissues enjoy periods of rest between impulses and longer rest periods when the activator is out of the mouth, as is usual for the greater proportion of the 24 hours. The result of this cycle of impulse and resting phase is thought to be a lessening of possible ill effects on the tooth roots and periodontal tissues, tooth movement by activators being characterized by a maintenance of normal periodontal thickness throughout the period of tooth movement (Häupl, Grossmann, and Clarkson, 1952).

THE DESIGN AND CONSTRUCTION OF FUNCTIONAL APPLIANCES

The functional appliance as originally designed was a loose-fitting appliance inserted between the teeth, lying against them at selected points and also making contact with the palate and soft tissues covering the inner side of the mandibular alveolar processes. Through these means functional stimuli were brought to bear on the teeth and through the teeth on the periodontal tissues, alveolar bone, and mandibular joint. What is sometimes not quite clear is whether the stimuli applied to the alveolar bone and mandibular joint result from pressures applied to the teeth only or whether it was originally intended to apply stimuli to the alveolar bone through its covering soft tissue also. It is noted by Häupl, Grossmann, and Clarkson, on the basis of clinical observation, that: "these appliances function even when no longer in contact with the teeth, since the latter had already changed position due to their influence. The results, therefore, were not due to the plate pressing on the teeth."†

---

* Quoted by kind permission of Arne Björk and *Sveriges Tandläkarförbunds Förlagsförening*, Stockholm.

† This and the quotation on p. 102 are by kind permission of William Grossmann and Henry Kimpton, London.

A fundamental practical and doctrinal consideration concerning the design and use of functional appliances is whether active or pressure elements should or should not be incorporated in the appliances. The principle of functional appliance design and use is that the appliances act through the functional stimuli applied to the teeth, alveolar bone, and remote parts of the dentofacial complex and through the guiding of the teeth during their normal eruption and growth paths. From the doctrinal point of view the addition of active parts to the appliances may be regarded as an illogical complication of the clear, fundamental principle of functional stimulation (Watry, 1947). From the purely practical point of view, the addition of active parts to a functional appliance creates technical difficulties in construction and adjustment, and the required looseness of the appliance may lead to imprecision in the application of individual pressures to teeth or may impair the proper functioning of the activator. As, however, teeth may be moved by active pressures, and the vast majority of tooth movements are carried out in this way, if active parts can be incorporated in functional appliances without reducing the efficiency of the appliance as a functional device, there seems to be no real objection to the combination of the two methods of treatment within the same appliance. The true objections to such an amalgamation lie in the possibility that an appliance may be produced that is neither functionally nor actively effective.

The degree to which the scope of a functional appliance may be extended and elaborated by the addition of active parts must lie with the designer and user of the appliance, and when the combination of functional and active pressures in the same appliance becomes too complicated to be efficient, discretion will rule that treatment should be broken down into stages and either active appliances or functional appliances used, depending on the nature of the tooth movements required.

THE ANDRESEN APPLIANCE

The Andresen appliance or monobloc is probably the most frequently used of the activator group of appliances because of the dramatically successful treatment of Class II, div. 1 malocclusion that it can effect in some cases. In such cases the true idea of the monobloc as a functional appliance holds good for the reason that the appliance is designed to fit the occlusion only when the mandible and lower dentition are in a forward, functional position and the muscular effort used to bring the mandible to its position of centric relation produces the pressures which determine the morphological changes which ensue. (*Fig.* 161.)

The use of the monobloc to produce changes in other directions, either a distal shifting of the lower dentition in relation to the upper or changes in lateral direction, is fraught with difficulties which do not arise where the treatment of postnormal occlusion is concerned.

In Class III malocclusion it is not easy to produce such definite functional pressures in the desired directions as it is possible to produce in postnormal occlusion because the mandible cannot be displaced distally in the same way as it can be displaced forward. The forward position of the mandible used in the functional treatment of postnormal occlusion is a functional position for which there is no equivalent functional distal position in Class III malocclusion, a position which would be available for the functional treatment of this malrelationship. In the circumstances the best that can be done is to construct an activator which is split horizontally, the two parts being connected by a horizontally working screw which, when opened, displaces the two portions of the appliance, the lower part distally, the upper mesially by small degrees. When worn as a functional appliance, mesial pressure on the upper teeth and distal on the lower can be brought to bear only when the opposing upper and lower dentitions are brought together in a vertical direction by the muscles of mastication, through the action of inclined planes in the activator.

The limitations of the activator in the treatment of Class III malocclusion are emphasized by the inclusion in the appliance used in such treatment, by most authorities, of arches or springs intended to bring about proclination of the upper labial segment and retroclination

105

of the teeth in the lower labial segment. Such limited tooth movements in any case often constitute the sole treatment of certain Class III malocclusions, and it may be that these movements could be more effectively carried in the first instance. In restricting the use of the appliance in this way many advantages are to be obtained in that, under favourable circumstances, only one appliance may need to be used, inspections and adjustments may be

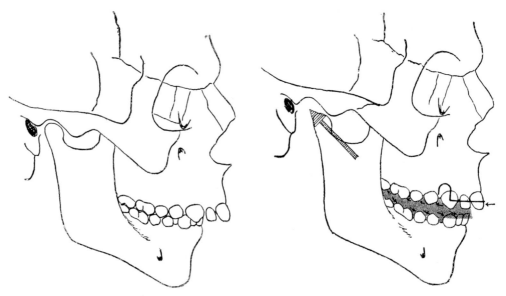

Fig. 161.—The main backward pull of the muscles of mastication is transferred to the teeth individually through the Andresen plate. The upper teeth are pushed in a distal direction, the lower teeth in a mesial direction.

out by appliances other than the activator equipped with auxiliary bows and springs.

In the treatment of discrepancies in the occlusion in a bucco-lingual direction, again certain problems are to be found in connexion with the use of activator appliances. It is sometimes suggested that different degrees of growth may be brought about in the condyle heads by taking the working bite for an activator with the mandible to one side, so leading to the correction of cross-bite conditions by the wearing of an activator constructed to such a bite. In the treatment of such conditions, however, means are usually shown for producing buccal movement of upper teeth and lingual movement of lower teeth by means of auxiliary attachments on activator appliances.

The success of the Andresen appliance in the treatment of straightforward Class II, div. 1 malocclusions is a strong recommendation for using the activator only in cases of this kind

carried out at relatively infrequent intervals, and at the end of treatment the appliance may simply be discarded or worn once or twice a week for two or three months before being discarded. Treatment may be completed within six to twelve months in favourable cases.

The term 'straightforward Class II, div. 1 malocclusion' is difficult to define, although what is intended may be comprehensible. The most important considerations are that the dental arches should be well arranged—that is to say, arranged in smooth curves without crowding or impactions in consequence of early loss of deciduous teeth; the upper labial segment may be proclined and spaced, the occlusal relation may be disturbed to the extent of a full unit anteroposteriorly, the overbite may be considerably increased.

Circumstances which indicate doubt as to the advisability of using the Andresen appliance include irregularities of the dental arches following early loss of deciduous teeth or due to disproportion in the size of the teeth and the size of the jaws; breaks in the dental arch following extraction of permanent teeth; open bite due to digit sucking or anomalies of function of the tongue or lips which persist through and after orthodontic treatment; inability of the lips to lie easily in contact when at rest. Such signs suggest difficulties in treatment and are warning signs as to the ultimate stability of the arrangement of the teeth produced in orthodontic treatment by any appliance method. Such signs indicate that the functional appliance may not be the most suitable apparatus for producing the kinds of tooth rearrangement that are looked for.

It is often advocated that very early treatment of postnormal occlusion using the activator, that is to say, in the deciduous dentition, brings benefits that are not available if treatment is delayed until the permanent dentition is in position. The suggested advantage of beginning treatment very early is that between the time of completion of the deciduous dentition and the accession of the permanent teeth lies a period of intense growth and developmental activity in the face, jaws, and dentition, and in such conditions the functional type of appliance could be expected to be more effective in directing the development of the occlusion than at a later age. This is theoretically true, and if a number of other important considerations are favourable there is everything to be said for giving the patient the advantages that may accrue from the utilization of as large a part of the most active growing period of the jaws and dentition as possible. The drawbacks to the very early commencement of orthodontic treatment are that the period of treatment and supervision becomes correspondingly prolonged, with consequent strain on the patient's interest and co-operation; the prolonged wearing of appliances brings its own problems in connexion with side-effects arising out of oral hygiene difficulties; the changeover from deciduous to permanent dentition may necessitate a series of new appliances; the occurrence of early loss of deciduous teeth may involve a complicated

appliance routine for the patient if space retention and active treatment are continued simultaneously; the later discovery of crowding, when the teeth in the labial segments eventually erupt, may be an unwelcome manifestation, necessitating a revision of the original diagnosis and plan of treatment.

Factors such as these, operating singly or in combination at different times over a prolonged period, can embarrass the course of treatment or nullify the possible benefits of commencing treatment at an early age. There is no clinical control in the individual case to show that early treatment necessarily confers the benefits of a more complete or more stable correction of the occlusal relationship than would be achieved by treatment later on, and it is a known fact that permanent dentitions, complete to the second molar teeth, exhibiting severe degrees of postnormal occlusion, can be quite easily treated by functional appliances to stable, normal occlusal relationship at the age of 11–12 years or older.

The age at which functional treatment of Class II, div. 1 malocclusion is commenced will be decided in the light of the foregoing considerations.

THE CONSTRUCTION OF THE ANDRESEN APPLIANCE

The construction of a functional appliance, activator, monobloc, or Andresen appliance for the treatment of Class II, div. 1 malocclusion requires working models and a wax bite. The impressions for the models should be taken in an alginate impression material and the edges of the impressions should extend to the limits of the labial and lingual sulci. It is important to see that the impression extends adequately into the lingual sulcus in the molar region in the lower denture and in the labial sulcus in the upper arch. Impressions that are short in these regions create unnecessary difficulties in the laboratory stages of appliance construction.

As starting points for the making of working bites for the treatment of Class II, div. 1 malocclusions the following details should be observed:—

1. The mandible should be brought forward until the buccal occlusal relationship is normal anteroposteriorly.

107

2. The bite should be open to a degree which separates the upper and lower labial segments, making it possible to cover the incisal edges of the lower incisors with the baseplate material of the appliance and leave

mandible. A horseshoe-shaped bite block is favoured and has the advantage of leaving the lingual area of the mouth free during the taking of the bite, but must be carefully handled during insertion and removal from the

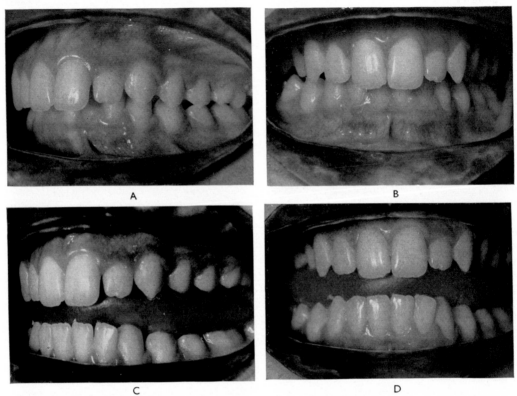

Fig. 162.—A, This patient has increased overbite and one unit postnormal occlusion. B, The teeth have been opened slightly to show that the centre lines of the upper and lower arches do not correspond. C, The bite for an Andresen appliance. The buccal segments are in normal relation anteroposteriorly. The bite has been opened sufficiently to separate the incisors. D, The centre lines in the working bite position are made to correspond.

room for modification of the appliance lingually to the upper incisors.

3. The centre lines should be made to correspond.

The working bite is taken in pink modelling wax, an adequate quantity of which is softened slightly and moulded to a convenient shape which may be varied according to the personal preferences of the operator. A solid transverse block of wax is less likely to become distorted during insertion and removal from the mouth, but may interfere unduly with the patient's tongue and cause difficulty in positioning the

mouth as it may easily become warped and hence difficult to place in an accurate position on the working models.

Some of the secrets of taking the working bite include the following points:—

Have enough wax in the block and have the main body of wax soft but firm; the surfaces may be flamed just before insertion to ensure a sharp impression of the occlusal surfaces of the teeth. The patient should have something definite to bite on and should not find a completely unresisting mass between the teeth.

The patient should be told what is expected of him and opening, protrusive, closing, and side-to-side movements rehearsed before putting in the bite block. When actually taking the bite, the patient is told to open, protrude the mandible, and close *very slowly* until told

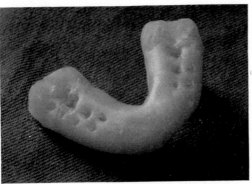

Fig. 163.—The wax bite for constructing the Andresen appliance.

to stop closing, at which point movement should stop with the mandible held quite still. The occlusal relationship can then be checked and any adjustment made by retrusion or sideways movement, without opening.

When the occlusal relationship is as required, a very small further closure may be made and the teeth immediately opened. The bite block should then be removed and chilled in cold water for a minute or so and replaced in the mouth, the patient carefully finding the position of occlusion in the wax. The teeth are then pressed into the wax with gentle firmness and opened. The teeth should come out of the wax with a slight click which indicates that the impression has been confirmed on the fully chilled wax. This second taking of the bite has the advantage of removing any small occlusal obstructions or warps that may have been introduced into the wax when removed from the mouth the first time (*Figs.* 162, 163).

The working models, which should be at hand, are placed in the working bite and firmly seated. At this stage the correctness and suitability of the bite relationship should be finally checked against the record models and the patient's occlusion. If all is correct the

models should be held in the working bite with a light elastic band and passed to the laboratory for construction of the appliance (*Fig.* 164).

As a rule it is not difficult to obtain the working bite for an activator. As the procedure

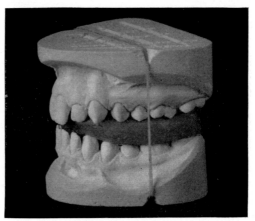

Fig. 164.—Working models placed in a wax bite held together by a light elastic band.

involves a voluntary action on the part of the patient, it is useful to consider patients and their reactions as falling into three categories:—

1. The sensible, intelligent patient who understands what is required and can produce any bite relationship that may be required. With such patients the bite may be taken in a moment.

2. The patient who misunderstands what is required but who is over-anxious to help. In such cases much time may be taken up with a large number of incorrect bites and completely spoiled bite blocks. The more the problem is explained, the more difficult it appears to be to achieve what is required from the patient.

3. The patient who does not understand what is required and who appears unable to carry out any of the movements requested. In such cases it may be possible for the operator to move the mandible into the required position and this may be the best that can be achieved, although with such a low degree of co-operation and understanding on the part of the patient the whole question of treatment with functional appliances in such cases should be carefully considered.

8

There are very few cases in which serious difficulty arises in taking a bite for the construction of a functional appliance.

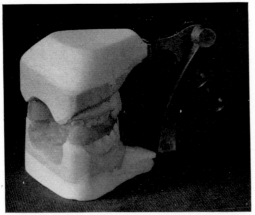

Fig. 165.—Models have been placed on plane-line articulator. The blades of the articulator are parallel.

LABORATORY PROCEDURES

An Andresen appliance by tradition is a baseplate which fits both the upper and lower dentitions, with a simple bow which maintains control of the teeth in the upper labial segment.

The construction of such an appliance falls naturally into the following stages: articulating the models; construction of the labial bow; waxing the baseplates; inserting the labial bow; joining the baseplates together; flasking, packing, and finishing.

Articulating the Models.—The easiest way of articulating the models is to use a standard, plane-line articulator with the incisor teeth facing towards the hinge of the articulator. The lingual aspect of the models faces outwards and this greatly facilitates the waxing up of the baseplate (*Fig.* 165). It is important to have the bases of the models cut down enough to permit the insertion of the models with the intervening working bite between the blades or forks of the articulator when they are parallel. It is then possible to withdraw the models from the articulator without separating them from the working bite or from the waxed-up appliance when this later stage is finished. The possibility of removing the models from the articulator in this way avoids

damage to the articular surfaces of the models which might occur if the articulated models are simply opened from the wax bite

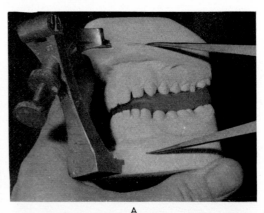

A

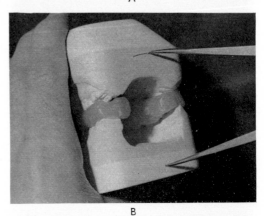

B

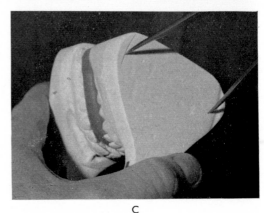

C

Fig. 166.—The height of the bite is registered: A, Anteriorly; B, Posteriorly; C, The recording is registered on the base of the models.

or from the waxed-up appliance. If the models are taken off the articulator together they may be separated from the wax bite by slight warming, if necessary, and the waxed appliance may be gently eased off the working models separately prior to flasking and

thinner wire will be required if pressure is to be exerted on the upper incisor teeth by compressing the U-loops, as bows of the kind described are always relatively stiff and it is difficult to obtain sensitive control of the amount of pressure exerted by bows made of rather thick

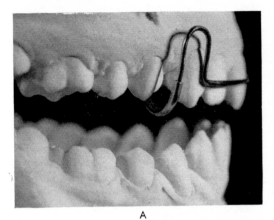 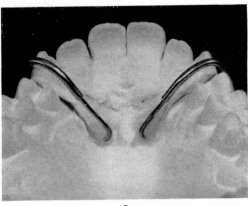

A   B

Fig. 167.—A, The labial bow of 0·8-mm. wire is reinforced with stainless steel tubing where it will enter the baseplate. Note that the tag of the bow runs well clear of the upper canine and premolar teeth. B, The tags of the labial bow are turned down at right angles to the palate. This simple attachment is perfectly satisfactory.

finishing the appliance. When the models are fixed on the articulator the setting screw is locked, and as a further precaution the vertical dimension between the models is measured and registered on the bottom of the lower model before the models are disturbed from their positions in the wax bite (*Fig.* 166).

Construction of the Labial Bow.—The models are removed from the articulator and freed from the wax bite and from any particles of wax that may be adhering to them.

A plain labial bow is then constructed for the upper model extending distally to the centres of the labial surfaces of the canine teeth and with a U-loop at either side. The ends of the bow pass between the canine and first premolar teeth into the palate. The bow should be made of a robust gauge of hard stainless steel wire of about 0·9-mm. thickness. If a more resilient bow is required, a thickness of 0·8 mm. may be used, in which case it is advisable to reinforce the wire at the point where it enters the baseplate by sliding on a short length of annealed stainless steel tube of the correct internal diameter (*Fig.* 167). The

wires. The labial bow as described is used to cause the teeth in the labial segment to follow the movement of the teeth in the buccal segments as changes in the occlusal relation take place. The bow may also be activated a little to produce a lingual inclination of the teeth in the labial segment.

When bringing the ends of the labial bow through into the palate of the upper model it is important to keep the wire clear of the teeth and to make the tags pass equidistantly between the upper and lower rows of teeth. Sometimes the tags are brought through to the palate in contact with the embrasure between the upper canine and first premolar teeth. In consequence, when the appliance is later trimmed with a steel bur there is danger of damaging the wire as it lies near the surface of the baseplate material. If the wire is passed midway between the upper and lower teeth it is deep within the baseplate material in this situation and the risk is less of cutting as far down as the wire when trimming the appliance.

The final anchorage of the ends of the labial bow in the baseplate can be quite simple, and

111

if the tips of the ends are turned down against the palate this will ensure that the tag is held securely in the baseplate material. When the labial bow is finished it is laid aside in readiness for inserting into the upper baseplate.

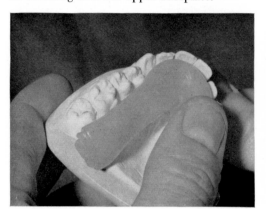

Fig. 168.—The softened roll of wax is placed just below the occlusal surfaces of the teeth.

Waxing the Baseplates.—This should be done in the following stages:—

1. Wax up the upper and lower baseplates.
2. Insert the labial bow in the upper baseplate.
3. Join the baseplates together with the models on the articulator.
4. Smooth off the waxing of the complete appliance.

When the time comes to transform the wax prototype of the appliance into acrylic material this may be done in one of two ways. Either the wax may be sealed to the working casts on which it was constructed and models and wax embedded in the flask for completion of the packing and polymerizing procedures; or the wax image of the appliance may be removed from the plaster casts on which it was constructed and embedded in the flask by itself and subsequently converted into an acrylic reproduction.

The second procedure is the simpler of the two in many ways and more satisfactory, but it is essential that the wax prototype of the appliance should reproduce accurately the fitting surfaces of the teeth and gingival margins of the casts on which it was constructed, and great care must be taken to ensure that the

wax pattern is not allowed to warp between its removal from the articulator and its final, secure embedding in the laboratory flask.

In waxing-up the upper and lower baseplates, therefore, it is essential to see that the wax is

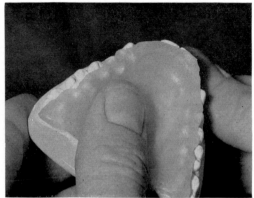

Fig. 169.—The wax is pressed firmly into the embrasures between the teeth and spread down into the palate.

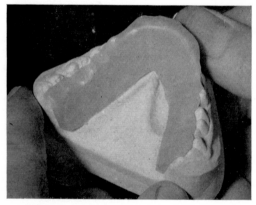

Fig. 170.—The lower baseplate waxed up from a roll of softened wax. Note that the incisal edges of the front teeth are capped with a thin layer of wax.

soft enough to take a good impression of the embrasures between the lingual aspects of the teeth.

The recommended procedure is to wet the dental casts in fairly warm water, but not to soak the plaster so long that free water remains lying on the surface when the models are left for a few moments in the air. The wetting and slight warming of the casts have two objects: First, well-softened wax will not stick to the

112

damp surface; and, secondly, the slightly warm plaster will not chill the surface of the warm, soft wax and hence prevent it from spreading closely into the gingival crevices.

For the purpose of adapting the wax to the tooth surfaces and the adjoining gingiva it is better not to apply the wax as a sheet but in a roll about 1 cm. in diameter with a firmly soft centre and very well softened outer layer.

This roll is taken and curved to fit the dental arch lingually, lying just below the gum margin (*Fig.* 168). The top, very soft surface is then firmly pressed out against the teeth and into the embrasures between them and on to their occlusal surfaces (*Fig.* 169). This should be done at once rapidly right around the dental arch from one side to the other. Care must be taken in the incisor region not to break off any of the teeth. If the wax is soft, light but sufficient pressure employed, and, as a precaution, the incisor teeth supported on the labial side with a curved forefinger, there will be no danger of damaging the model.

In the lower model the softened wax should be taken up to and over the incisal edges of the front teeth in a thin layer. It is important to avoid putting a thick layer of hard wax over the lower incisors at this stage, as when the baseplates are subsequently pressed into contact a spot of excessive pressure may occur over the lower incisors, leading to fracture of the plaster teeth (*Fig.* 170).

When the wax has been safely adapted to the teeth and gum margins the remainder of the roll should be devoted to the construction of the baseplate areas of the upper and lower parts of the appliance. In the upper arch the wax may be stretched down into the palate and the segments from either side joined in the midline with a hot wax knife. It is important to avoid pulling the wax away from the teeth during this stage. If there is sufficient wax in the roll this method has the advantage that the upper part of the appliance is made in one piece of wax, and with a little care the line of fusion in the middle line can be completely obliterated. If there is surplus wax, the palate area should be scraped down to a suitable and uniform thickness and smoothed with the flame. If necessary, wax can be added to complete the construction of the palate.

An alternative method for the completion of the construction of the upper baseplate is as follows: When the wax has been well adapted to the teeth it may be scraped down from the lingual aspect until only what is essential to fit the teeth and gum margin is left, after which a palate may be added as a fresh single layer of softened wax. With this method it may be difficult to avoid leaving a noticeable line of junction between the two wax applications when the appliance is seen from the palatal aspect, and in scraping down the first application of wax great care must be exercised to avoid going too far and taking a cut off an underlying tooth.

In the lower arch the wax roll is usually sufficient to complete the construction of the baseplate; the available wax is simply pressed down into the lingual sulcus and trimmed to shape.

Inserting the Labial Bow.—The simplest method for placing the labial bow in the upper

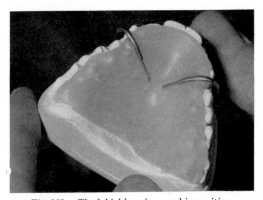

Fig. 171.—The labial bow is waxed in position.

baseplate is to try on the bow to find exactly where it fits in the baseplate and then to soften the appropriate area of the baseplate with a hot knife sufficiently to tack in the bow precisely in its required position. The softened spot of wax is cooled with an air stream and the bow securely fastened with pink wax flowed around the tags. The method of heating the tags of the bow and melting them into the baseplate is clumsy and liable to be inaccurate

113

as it is difficult to heat the tags to the right temperature for long enough to give time to place the wire precisely. If the wire is not hot enough it will not melt the wax. If it is too hot an excessive amount of wax is melted and runs away, after which there is a delay while the wax cools enough to hold the wire; meanwhile, the bow must be held in place with great accuracy. The fact that the recommended fitting of the tags requires that they do not lie against the plaster but only touch at their bent-down ends, means that the bow can usually be held in position by the turned-down tips for positioning purposes, after which the bow is properly secured with wax flowed around the tags, fastening them to the surface of the baseplate (*Fig.* 171).

Joining the Baseplates together.—The models are replaced on the articulator and the articulator closed. At this stage it is important to

The sealing together of the baseplates is done with a roll of very well-softened wax, the occlusal surfaces of the baseplates being carefully flamed just before inserting the roll and closing the articulator.

When the articulator is being closed a check should be made on the vertical dimension between the upper and lower models, using the registration marks and recorded dimension originally provided. Care should be taken to see that the articulator is closed as far as, but not beyond, the original registration.

The waxing-up of the appliance is completed by smoothing off the joint between the upper and lower parts, attending to the fit and neatness of the waxing around the incisor segments, and smoothing the lingual surface of the appliance with a small, fine flame of the gas/air blowlamp. The wax is then thoroughly chilled in cold water or left in a cold atmosphere

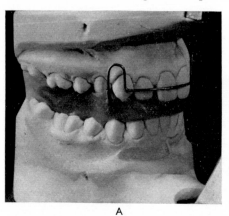 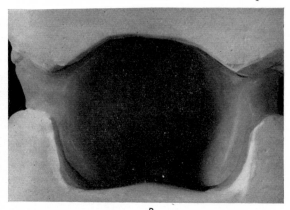

A   B

Fig. 172.—**A,** The completed waxed-up Andresen appliance. **B,** The lingual view of the Andresen appliance. Note that the lingual undercuts in the molar region of the lower model have been plastered out and that in this area the appliance is constructed with well-rounded flanges against which the tongue lies comfortably.

examine the occluding surfaces of the two plates to make quite sure that they do not actually touch, but that there is at least 1 mm. or more clearance between the wax overlying the occlusal and incisal surfaces of the teeth. The reason for this clearance is that, when softened wax is put between the models and the baseplates pressed together, there is a risk that if the baseplates touch at any point, excessive pressure may build up at this spot and lead to damage of the underlying plaster, particularly in the incisor area.

until cold right through. The models are removed together from the articulator and then each model is very carefully taken off the wax appliance. Final trimming of the appliance may then be carried out: the lateral flanges may be reduced to half the width of the teeth in the buccal segments as this will save considerable time and labour in cutting the finished appliance; the lingual flange of the lower part of the appliance can be trimmed to the correct depth and smoothed and rounded. No other trimming of the appliance should be

114

done at this stage. The models should then be finally seated in the appliance to ensure that no occlusal interferences have been introduced through the trimming of the buccal flanges, and the wax appliance is ready for flasking and finishing (*Fig.* 172).

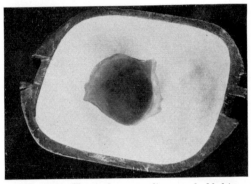

Fig. 173.—The Andresen appliance embedded in the deep half of the flask. The appliance is packed from the lingual side.

the flasking process a thin mix of the plaster investment should be brushed into the impression of the various tooth surfaces in the wax to ensure that air bubbles are not trapped, so causing failure of the appliance finally to fit. If the wax pattern is wetted with a 2 per cent solution of cetavlon, or a proprietary wetting agent, the consequent reduction in surface tension is a further insurance against the inclusion of air bubbles about the crevices of the tooth impressions in the wax.

This method of investment ensures that the fitting surface of the appliance is completely enveloped in one half of the flask so that risk of distorting the appliance is largely avoided. The second half of the flask is poured after applying separating medium to the lower half, When the plaster is set the flask is heated and the halves separated. The wax is washed out, the flask packed, and the baseplate material

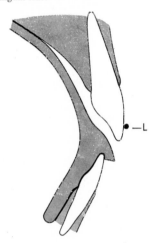

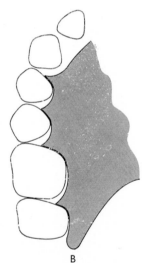

A   B

Fig. 174.—A, The trimming of the Andresen appliance in the incisor region. Baseplate material is removed behind the upper incisors well up to the apical region. The lower incisors remain capped in the baseplate. L, Labial bow. B, The trimming of the Andresen appliance in the upper buccal segments. Note that the appliance impinges on the mesial aspects of the premolar and molar teeth and is cut away behind the labial segment. In the lower arch the facets are made to touch the teeth in the buccal segments distally.

Flasking, Packing, and Finishing.—The wax model of the appliance is flasked upside down in the deep part of the flask with the plaster investment brought to the posterior edge of the palate and the lower edge of the lingual flange of the lower baseplate (*Fig.* 173). During

processed in the normal way. The acrylic materials in the normal pink colour are perfectly satisfactory for the construction of the kind of activator that is under discussion.

After processing and cooling, the appliance is deflasked, cleaned, and dried. Excess acrylic material, present as 'flash' around the lower and posterior edges, is removed and the appliance smoothed and polished to the shape of the wax pattern that was originally invested laboratory. Only if this is done can it be ensured that the bite of the appliance corresponds with the working bite taken originally for the patient. If the teeth do not meet evenly and

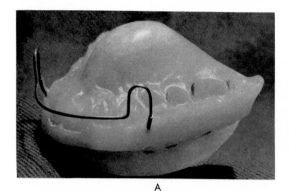 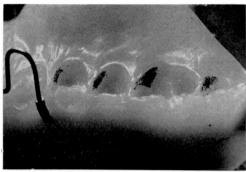

A B

Fig. 175.—A, The completed Andresen appliance. B, The areas intended as facets to impinge on the teeth in the buccal segments have been marked with lead pencil.

in the flask. At this stage the acrylic appliance is placed on the models which are returned to the articulator and the registration of vertical dimension finally checked. The appliance exactly in their impressions in the appliance, anteriorly and posteriorly, and there is any sign that the bite has been 'raised' or otherwise disturbed during the construction of the appliance, the appliance should be recon-

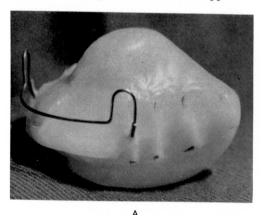 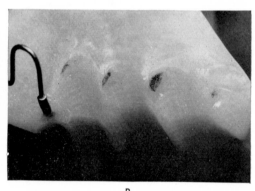

A B

Fig. 176.—A, The Andresen appliance after the left side has been trimmed in the incisor region and in the buccal segments. B, The pencil markings on the facets are still to be seen. Note the channels along which eruption of the teeth can take place.

should now fit the occlusion of the patient exactly with the mandible forward in the working bite position.

FITTING AND ADJUSTING OF THE ACTIVATOR

The activator is first of all placed in the mouth exactly as it is received from the structed as it never is possible to make an ill-fitting appliance fit satisfactorily by cutting or otherwise adjusting it.

Cutting the Monobloc.—If the appliance fits correctly it should then be cut to facilitate the tooth movements that are intended. The cutting of an Andresen appliance means that

116

baseplate material should be removed lingually to the upper incisors, distally to the teeth in the upper buccal segments, and mesially to the teeth in the lower buccal segments. The capping over the lower incisors

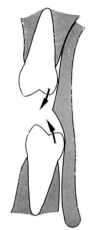

Fig. 177.—If required, the channels in which the buccal teeth lie are curved outwards, so guiding the eruption of these teeth and creating expansion of the arches.

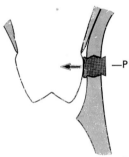

Fig. 179.—Buccal movement of a molar tooth by means of a pad of rubber pulled into an undercut hole in the baseplate. P, Rubber pad. The plug should project about 1–2 mm. against the tooth and should be cut off flush on the lingual side of the baseplate. The rubber used is separating rubber, which is obtainable in strips about ⅛ in. square in section.

should be left in position (Fig. 174). Trimming is best done with a steel bone bur in the straight handpiece, and if the facets which must be left in the buccal segments are marked with a soft lead pencil before cutting is started, the trimming may be done with great precision (Fig. 175). The channels which run between

the upper and lower teeth in the buccal segments should run downwards and backwards (Fig. 176). If it is intended that there should be expansion of the buccal segments, the channels in the appliance may be constructed

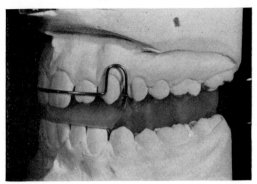

Fig. 178.—The trimmed Andresen appliance on the working models.

to guide the premolar and molar teeth buccally (Fig. 177). In these circumstances the buccal movement of the teeth can only take place if the teeth erupt farther. The effects of these trimming procedures are apparent in Fig. 178.

Any sharp edges left by the cutting of the appliance are smoothed off and all is ready for final trial of the appliance in the mouth.

CASE REPORT

A. C., aged 12 years (Figs. 179, 180).

DIAGNOSIS.—Dental base relation a little postnormal. Upper lip a little short, lower lip postures lingually to the upper incisors. The dental arches were complete with the permanent teeth to the first permanent molars, the upper incisors were proclined and spaced, the lower incisors were well alined. The lower buccal segments were one unit postnormal to the upper, the overbite was increased and complete. 6| occluded lingually to 6|.

TREATMENT.—A Sved plate was worn for three months as an experiment in patient co-operation. The overbite was reduced and there was a slight improvement in the occlusal relation. An Andresen appliance was then fitted. Cephalometric X-rays and record models were made. Eighteen months later the occlusal relation was correct anteroposteriorly. The incisor relation had improved very greatly. The relationship of 6| to 6| was corrected by means of a rubber plug pulled into the appliance lingually to 6| (Hopkin, 1958) (Fig. 179). A Hawley retainer with inclined plane was fitted and worn for six months. Final records were taken one year after completion of the treatment with the Andresen appliance.

Table V details the cephalometric measurements before and after treatment. From this it can be seen that SNA–SNB difference had hardly changed. The upper incisors were retroclined by 22°, the lower incisors proclined 6°. Both upper and lower prognathism was slightly less after than before treatment.

117

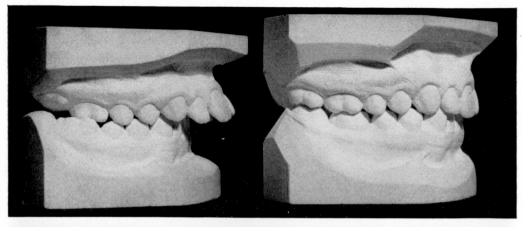

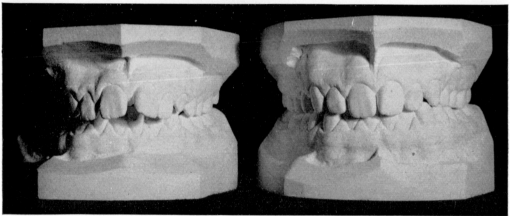

Fig. 180.—Postnormal occlusion. Class II, division 1 case treated with an Andresen appliance. A, Before treatment; B, After treatment.

THE FUNCTION CORRECTOR

The Function Corrector, sometimes referred to as the "Vestibular Appliance" or the "Fränkel Appliance", was originated by Dr. Rolf Fränkel of Zwickau, East Germany, about the middle of the present century.

The basic theoretical principle underlying the mode of action of this appliance is the idea that within the jaws and dento-alveolar processes there is, at practically every site, the possibility of bone deposition and resorption, especially during the growing period. It is further held that the amounts and directions

Table V.—Cephalometric Analysis

	SNA	SNB	SNA–SNB DIFFERENCE	$\underline{1|1}$ TO SN	$\overline{1|1}$ TO MANDIBULAR PLANE
Before	78·0°	74·5°	3·5°	122°	89°
After	76·0°	73·0°	3·0°	100°	95°
Difference	−2·0°	−1·5°	−0·5°	−22°	+6°

118

of bone deposition are influenced by variations in the pressure environment of the jaws and alveolar processes brought about by the posture and activity of the tongue, lips, and cheeks. The function corrector therefore seeks to modify the soft tissue positions and activities and thereby to influence the amounts and directions of bone deposition that are taking place within the dento-alveolar complex.

Function correctors are skeleton mouth shields which lie in the vestibule of the mouth and stand clear of all portions of the dento-alveolar system which are under-developed. The wire elements unite the lateral shields with the lip pads and serve also as guiding, stabilizing and "reflex inducing" factors.

It is from the physical nature of the appliance and its theoretical mode of action that the appliance derives its name, "The Vestibular Appliance or Function Corrector".

The following extract[*] from the writings of Dr. Fränkel embodies what appear to be the main theoretical principles which underlie the mode of action of the appliance and determine its application to the treatment of various kinds of irregularities and malocclusions.

Configuration and structure of the toothbearing gnathic skeleton are subject to mechanical influences of the environment which have the effect of modifying the growth sites and leading to the formation of a supporting structure. Such mechanical modification and activation of the growth sites may be due to the following four types of factors:—

1. Mechanical factors which are associated with the development, i.e., the influence of growth-linked changes in the size and shape of skeletal and environmental soft tissues.

2. Mechanical factors of a functional nature, i.e., the influence of physical functions such as oral seal, mastication, deglutition, play of features, respiration and so on.

3. The mechanical potential of the atmospheric pressure which by acting on the soft tissue mass is responsible, to a considerable extent, for the mechanical situation in the gnathic region.

4. The potential of the force of gravity, which exerts its influence especially on the tongue and the mandible.

It should therefore be the chief aim of orthodontic therapy to trace and eliminate any abnormal mechanical potentials in the environmental soft tissues. Mechanical factors of a functional nature are the most serious of those mentioned above, and any dysfunction or complete absence of oral seal deserves our closest attention.

In dealing with this we should bear in mind the fact

that a physiologically normal oral seal is only ensured if three requirements are fulfilled:—

1. Anterior oral seal, brought about by lip seal with normal tension.

2. Posterior oral seal, brought about by the contact between soft palate and root of the tongue.

3. Median oral seal, brought about by the contact between dorsum of the tongue and hard palate.

In this connexion I would refer to the investigations made by Donders (1953), Körbitz (1914), Noltemeier (1949), Eckert-Möbius (1962), and Fränkel (1964). According to these authors, the natural rest position of the tongue against the roof of the palate is not due to muscular action but is maintained solely by the action of the atmospheric pressure. Their investigations revealed that the deglutition reflex, which is accompanied by lip seal, results in the air being "pumped out" of the cavum proprium by the tongue's peristalsis, thus creating a partial vacuum which is completely filled by the soft tissue of the tongue, under the action of the atmospheric pressure. In this way we get a completely enclosed space between tongue on the one hand and lips and cheeks on the other hand. This space must be regarded as the most appropriate site for directing the morphogenesis of the toothbearing alveolar process.

But the above-mentioned environmental mechanical factors and their importance for the morphogenesis and configuration of the gnathic skeleton should not be interpreted in terms of functional influences alone. The neuromotor functions of respiration, food intake and digestion are not acquired, like motor functions, but are congenital, that is to say, they are perfect from birth owing to the unconditioned-reflex control mechanism. This functional mechanism therefore is a hereditary feature. Moreover, the individual and hereditary characteristics become clearly evident in the play of the features and in this respect one may say that, given a normal environment, its mechanical influences assume the quality of genetic information. Thus the genotypical arrangement of the soft tissue and its neuromotor functions affords an excellent explanation for all cases of striking family likeness. But as the phenotype invariably constitutes a combination of hereditary and environmental factors the appearance of orofacial soft tissue and especially the play of the features should not be taken merely as the result of a hereditary disposition. They should also be regarded as the reflection of the individual's psychic development, which results from his confrontation with the environment. This is the background which gave rise to our optimistic view that any soft-tissue atypia will be amenable to functional treatment.

If we subscribe to the principle of a "proper education of the jaw", an analysis of the above will show that the first and foremost object of orthodontics should be a normalization of the environment of the growing jaw. Our therapeutic measures should chiefly be directed at eliminating any atypical features in the three-fold oral seal and acquired habits, especially any abnormal functioning of the perioral muscles during deglutition. Normalization of the oral seal also creates the main prerequisites for a normalization of respiration. Teleradiographic examinations showed that this kind of treatment resulted frequently in a significant dilatation of the epipharynx and recession of the swelling of the nasopharyngeal tonsil.

[*] This extract from the *Transactions* of the *European Orthodontic Society*, 1966, is reproduced by kind permission of Dr. Rolf Fränkel and the Editor.

The function corrector has been shown to be an effective appliance for the treatment of malocclusions of certain kinds and where such malocclusions are encountered the use of the function corrector should be considered. Malocclusions of the Class II, division 1 and Class III type and anterior open bite have reacted favourably to treatment in the author's experience. It is therefore proposed to discuss the design and construction of the appliance in a number of varieties and to include case histories of successfully and unsuccessfully treated subjects.

Design and Construction of the Function Corrector.—There are three types of Function Corrector.

Type I Function Corrector or F.R.1.—This type is used in the treatment of Angle Class I and Class II, division 1 malocclusions.

The lower lip shields are supports for the lower lip and prevent the action of the mentalis muscle in producing pressure on the lower incisors. The action of the lower lip shields is valuable in situations where there is retroclination or crowding of the lower incisors whether the occlusion as a whole is normal or postnormal.

The buccal shields relieve pressure on the lateral aspects of the dental arches which leads to expansion, especially in the upper arch.

In Class II, division 1 cases the lower lip shield has the function of encouraging the adoption of a forward position of the lower lip which embraces the shield on effecting lip closure.

The action of the U loops in the lingual bow is important in the reduction of distocclusion. If the lower jaw slips back from the protruded position in which the regulator is made, the U loops on the lingual bow make contact with the mucous membrane on the lingual surface on the lower anterior alveolar tissues, thereby initiating a reflex which encourages the lower jaw to adopt the forward position.

In the treatment of postnormal occlusion, whether division 1 or 2, a forward positioning of the lower jaw in taking the functional bite is necessary.

The F.R.1 appliance is also used in the treatment of open bite. When used for this purpose, Fränkel advises that lip pads should be placed below both the upper and the lower

lips and states that it is not necessary to place any screen or wire to limit the projection of the tongue between the incisor teeth.

Type II Function Corrector or F.R.2.—This is used for treatment of Class II, division 2 malocclusion, and retroclination of the upper incisors is dealt with by a lingual arch in the upper part of the appliance behind the upper incisors; activation of this arch will produce proclination of these teeth. Otherwise, the action of the corrector is the same as in Class II, division 1 types of cases, in that the labial pads at the lower incisors relieve pressure of the lower lip on the lower incisors, and the correct occlusal relation is established by the bite with which the appliance is made.

Type III Function Corrector or F.R.3.—In this type the pressure of the upper lip on the upper incisors is relieved by pads which are placed over the upper alveolar process, and the action of the labial bow on the lower part of the appliance has the effect of correcting the incisor relationship, if necessary, by the retroclination of the lower incisors.

CONSTRUCTION OF THE FUNCTION CORRECTOR

Clinical Procedures.—

1. *Preparation of Dental Casts.*—Impressions are taken in alginate material of the upper and lower dental arches and adjacent tissues. The impressions must extend to the full depth of the buccal and lingual sulci and cover the palate to the posterior limit of the hard palate. The impressions are poured in a hard or stone plaster and the working casts should be at hand when the bite is being taken.

2. *Taking the Bite.*—An adequate roll of softened pink wax is used and the nature of the bite registration will vary with the type of malocclusion being treated. The molar part of the bite must be adequately registered. (*Fig.* 181.)

Class I malocclusion: The bite is taken with the incisors edge-to-edge and in contact.

Class II malocclusion (divisions 1 and 2): In taking the bite the mandible is moved forward to bring the buccal segments into a normal anteroposterior relationship and the teeth are closed together until contact is established.

120

The amount by which the mandible is moved forward is influenced also to some extent by the overjet and overbite and inclination of the incisor segments. The comfort of the patient when wearing the appliance must be considered

if the sulcus is deepened artificially too much the labial pads which result can easily be trimmed to prevent irritation of the labial sulcus, but pads which are too shallow cannot easily be added to at a later stage.

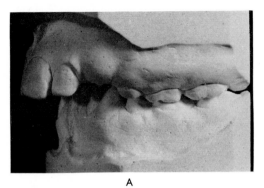
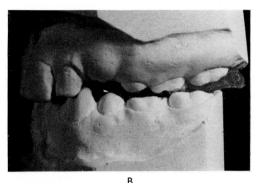

A   B

Fig. 181.—Construction of the function regulator. Taking the bite. A, Postnormal occlusion. B, The mandible is brought forward and the teeth brought together into contact.

and to bring the mandible too far forward will mean that the appliance will not be worn.

Class III malocclusion: The bite is taken as nearly as possible with the incisors edge-to-edge, no protrusion of the mandible being allowed. It is sometimes advisable not to close the teeth fully together into contact if the lower incisors overlap the upper to any marked degree and, when constructing the appliance, to place biting blocks between the upper and lower buccal segments attached to the buccal screens. Such biting planes or blocks prop the bite open sufficiently to allow the upper incisors to procline without the obstruction of the lower incisor teeth. If the lower incisor teeth do not overlap the uppers it is not usually necessary to put bite propping planes in the buccal segments.

3. *Adjustment of the Lower Dental Cast for F.R.1.*—The lower labial sulcus on the working model is compared with the appearance of the sulcus clinically. The working cast is trimmed with a round vulcanite cutter to ensure that the sulcus is sufficiently deep. If the impression does not record the full depth of the labial sulcus in the lower incisor region the labial pads when constructed will not hold the lower lip away from the lower incisor teeth. Even

Laboratory Procedures.—The following notes apply to the construction of a F.R.1 Appliance.

1. The working casts are mounted on a plain articulator using the working wax bite.

2. In the buccal segments wax of the thickness of 1·5 mm. is placed over the buccal segments of the teeth and the adjacent muscle covering of the alveolar process. When the buccal screens are subsequently constructed they will then be clear of the teeth and soft tissues.

3. The wire work, consisting of the following parts, is constructed in 0·9-mm. hard stainless-steel wire (*Fig.* 182 A–D):—

a. Palatal arch with central U loop. This arch must stand clear of the palate by 1–2 mm. and pass buccally between the occlusal surfaces of the cheek teeth. The ends of the archwire are formed into loops for anchorage in the buccal shields and then brought towards the midline to make rests lying on the occlusal surface of the upper second deciduous molars. If these teeth are not present the rests should lie upon the first permanent molars.

b. Upper labial arch with U loops opposite canine teeth.

c. Upper canine rests. These incorporate U loops palatally to the canine teeth.

121

d. It is recommended by Fränkel that the lower lingual arch be made in 0·9-mm. soft wire. It has been found in practice that hard wire may be used and that arches made of hard wire do not become distorted or broken.

e. Wire work for labial pads. This can be made in one piece but it is quicker and easier to use three pieces of wire for this part.

6. The resin may be allowed to cure at room temperature but this may allow porosity to develop. Curing of the resin may be accelerated by the use of a hydraulic pressure flask filled with lukewarm water. To get the

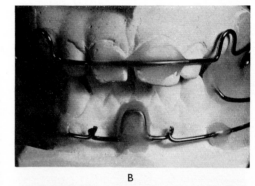

B

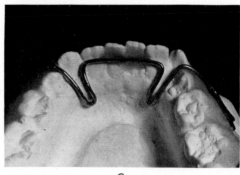

C

A

Fig. 182.—Construction of the wire assembly of the function corrector. A, The casts are placed on an articulator, the buccal segments are covered with a layer of wax, and the wire parts are prepared. B, The upper and lower labial bows. C, The lower lingual arch with loops. D, The upper labial bow and the palatal arch with central loop and occlusal rests. E, The clear acrylic screens have been built up by the technique for using quick curing acrylic material described in Chapter III. F, The complete appliance with the resin polymerized. G, H, I, The appliance trimmed down, polished, and replaced upon the dental casts.

All the wires are attached to the casts with hard wax at points which will not subsequently interfere with the application of the cold curing resin. All the tag ends of the wires are brought buccally for anchorage in the buccal shields.

4. The articulator is closed and the buccal wax padding made good at the line of the occlusion. A separating medium is applied to the plaster where the labial pads are to be constructed.

5. Cold curing clear acrylic material is used to build up the buccal wings and labial pads. (*Fig.* 182 E.)

appliance easily into the flask, the casts are removed together from the articulator and their bases cut down as much as necessary by means of a model grinder.

Using a hydraulic flask the resin sets rapidly, is free of porosity, and the heat involved is not enough to soften the wax and disturb the relative positions of the casts. (*Fig.* 182 F.)

7. When the resin has set all the wax is removed from the casts with hot water.

8. The appliance is trimmed and polished. (*Fig.* 182 G, H, I.)

9. An F.R.3 appliance is shown in *Fig.* 183.

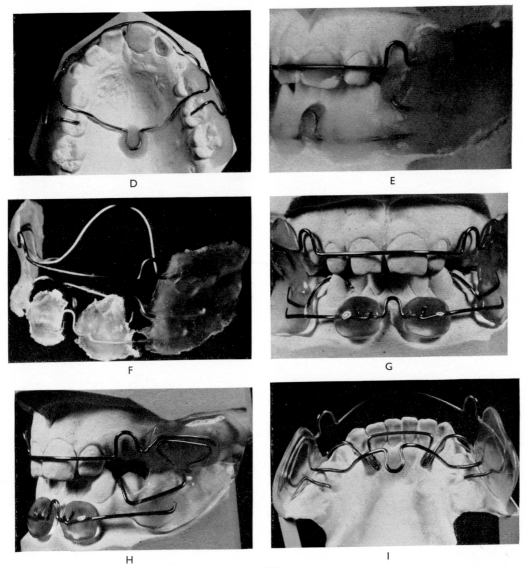

Fig. 182.

MANAGEMENT OF THE APPLIANCE

When the appliance is fitted the patient will be able to say at once whether there are any spots of discomfort or excessive pressure on teeth or soft tissues. Any such defects must be removed by adjusting the wire work or easing the acrylic material away from the labial mucosa. Pressure points under the screens or pads show as areas of blanching visible through the clear resin. The labial pads will, of course, lie against the alveolar mucosa when the appliance is first fitted and it is necessary to trim away an even thickness of from 1 mm. to 2 mm. from the alveolar surface of the pads. The depth to which the pads project into the labial sulcus must be carefully watched and, if there is any irritation of the mobile mucosa, the pads should be trimmed back at the offending spot and the trimmed surface polished.

123

Most patients will be able to wear the appliance full-time from the very first visit and to carry on a normal daily routine, apart from eating, with the appliance in place.

A patient who is self-conscious may for an initial period of a fortnight wear the appliance only on coming home from school and at night. Thereafter it must be worn at all times except

2. Prenormal occlusion (2 cases).

3. Anterior open bite (1 case).

The postnormal occlusions treated were all of the Class II, division 1 type and, as will be recognized, this includes a great many variations in different features. Some further classification of this group of 16 cases was carried out as follows.

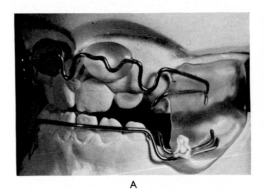
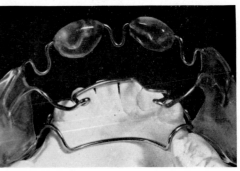

A   B

Fig. 183.—The F.R.3 appliance. A, The labial pads are lying under the upper lip and a labial bow lies against the lower incisors. B, Note that the lower lingual arch stands away from the lower incisors and alveolar process. There is an upper lingual arch which touches the upper incisors.

when eating. Very little maintenance or adjustment of the appliance is required apart from repair of accidental damage at the hands of the patient.

INDICATIONS FOR THE USE OF THE FUNCTION CORRECTOR*

The following set of case reports is the material of an investigation into indications for the use of functional correctors (Adams, 1969). The material for the report is a group of 19 cases which were treated with the Function Corrector. The cases were under treatment with the appliance for periods of from nine months to five years.

The presentation of 19 consecutive cases would not be feasible even if all had been successful, so that the material has been grouped in the following way:—

1. Postnormal occlusion (16 cases).

Subdivisions of Class II, Division I Malocclusion:—

1. Slight uncomplicated (2 cases).
2. Severe uncomplicated (5 cases).
3. With thumb sucking (4 cases).
4. With crowding (5 cases).
5. With early loss of deciduous teeth (3 cases).

Some cases came into more than one group and were therefore considered under more than one heading.

The postnormal occlusions and the open bite cases were treated with the F.R.1 type of appliance and the prenormal occlusions with the F.R.3. The results were as follows:—

Postnormal Occlusion
Good results   4 cases
No improvement   12 cases
Open Bite
Good result   1 case
Prenormal Occlusion
Good result   2 cases

Before discussing these results it is necessary to examine in more detail a few of the cases that were successfully treated and what occurred in them.

---

* The remainder of this chapter, from the heading "Indications for the Use of the Function Corrector" to the end, including all illustrations, is reproduced from the *Transactions of the European Orthodontic Society*, 1969, by kind permission of the Editor.

Postnormal Occlusion. —

The cases in question were:—

1. A girl in whom a severe malocclusion existed from the time of eruption of the deciduous dentition until the problem was treated with the F.R.1 at age 10 (category 2).

habits. Otherwise there was adequate room in the dental arches (category 2).

CASE REPORTS

1. *J. M.* (*Figs.* 184–7).—This patient attended aged 3 years 6 months with a history of lip sucking but not thumb sucking, although the appearance of the teeth strongly suggested a digit sucking habit. The patient's

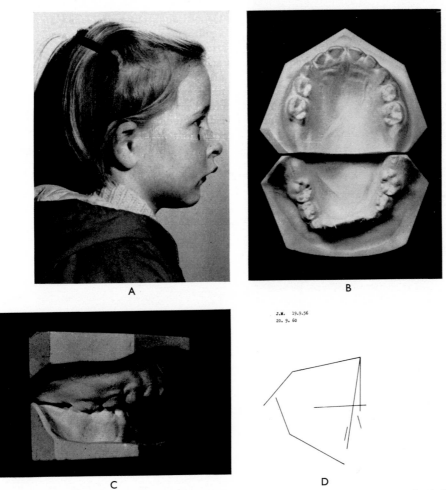

J.M.   19.9.56
20. 9. 60

Fig. 184.—J. M., aged 3 years 6 months. **A**, Profile. **B, C,** Dental casts. Note that in occlusal view the lower incisors appear to be pushed lingually, especially on the left, and the upper incisors are forward on the right. **D,** Tracing of cephalometric X-ray film.

2. Two boys in whom there was crowding of the dentition, early loss of deciduous teeth, and a severe postnormal occlusion (categories 4 and 5).

3. A boy of 3 years 2 months with a gross postnormal occlusion and with lip sucking

mother was emphatic that any thumb sucking that took place was very occasional. The subsequent treatment result confirmed that the digit habit was of no importance in this case and the parent's assessment was absolutely correct.

DIAGNOSIS.—A marked discrepancy in facial proportions was found with postnormality of the mandible and although the lips were of adequate proportions the lower lip lay continuously under the upper incisors and on

9

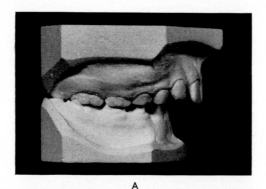

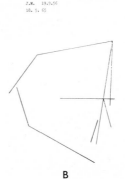

A

B

Fig. 185.—J. M., aged 8 years 8 months. **A**, Models, right view. **B**, Cephalometric tracing.

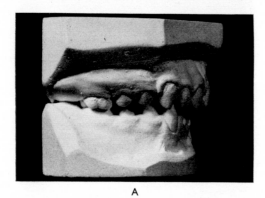

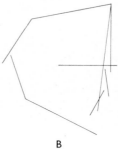

A

B

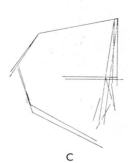

C

Fig. 186.—J. M., aged 11 years 2 months. **A**, Models, right view. **B**, Tracing at 11 years 2 months. **C**, Superimposition of tracings at 8 years 8 months and 11 years 2 months.

swallowing the lower lip contracted firmly against the tongue. (*Fig.* 184 **A**.)

A simple cephalometric analysis revealed that the SNA/B difference was high, 8°, lower incisors retroclined to 73° to mandibular plane, and the upper incisors proclined to 114·5° to the maxillary plane. There was a large overjet and incomplete, non-increased overbite. (*Fig.* 184 **B, C, D**.)

TREATMENT PLANNING.—The patient was so small and so young that no active treatment was initiated at this stage but yearly visits were instituted to observe growth progress and record by casts and cephalometric films the changes that were taking place.

At the age of 7 years the occlusion, facial pattern, and soft tissue activities were just as they had always been; the only difference was that permanent lower incisors were up instead of deciduous ones. (*Fig.* 185 **A, B**.) At this stage it was felt that something must be done to mitigate the condition and an attempt was made to aline the lower labial segment to a more forward position. The movement required being a simple proclination a removable appliance was used, but it was not possible to produce the tooth movement as planned: the teeth would not move but instead became mobile and it was deemed wiser after a short time not to continue with this line of treatment.

Subsequently an Andresen appliance was placed for a period of nine months at the age of 8 years, but as this treatment produced not the slightest change in the occlusion the appliance was abandoned. An oral screen

was also used for a short time but was also withdrawn quite soon.

Finally, it was decided that the Function Corrector might help the patient and at the age of 10 years the child was put on to Function Regulator treatment and within a few weeks improvements in the occlusal relationships began to take place. At the end of fourteen months, both upper and lower dental arch arrangement was

126

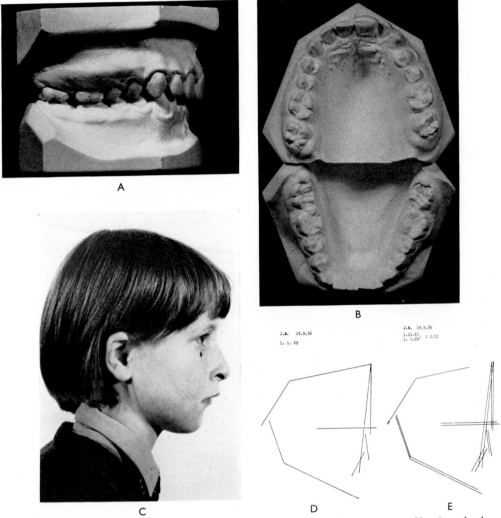

J.M. 19.9.56
1. 1. 69

J.M. 19.9.56
1.11.67) 1 2/12
1. 1.69)

Fig. 187.—J. M., aged 12 years 4 months. A, B, Models, right view and occlusal view. Note in occlusal view the symmetrical well arranged arches. C, Profile. Compare with *Fig.* 185. D, Tracing at 12 years 4 months. E, Superimposition of tracings at 11 years 2 months and 12 years 4 months.

excellent and incisor relationship was nearly normal, mainly due to proclination of the lower incisors, although the upper incisors had retroclined to some degree. (*Fig.* 186 A, B.)

The Fränkel appliance was continued for a further seven months, at the end of which time no further improvement in occlusal relationship had taken place and, as the molar relation was still postnormal, treatment was changed to the use of an Andresen appliance which produced some further occlusal improvement. The Andresen appliance was being worn until the age of 12 years 9 months. (*Fig.* 187 A, B, C, D, E.)

ASSESSMENT OF THE RESULT.—There is no doubt that in this case a rapid and dramatic improvement was made in the occlusion for this patient, although the appearance of the patient in profile does not appear greatly different before and after treatment as regards the relative prognathism of the upper and lower dental bases. The angle ANB at the end of treatment was 6°, a little less than the original 8° when the patient was first seen and 1° less than the 7° at the beginning of treatment. The mandible appears to have swung a little downward and forward during the time the patient has been under supervision and this may account for the change in ANB. The change in this angle of 2° appears to be due to an increase in the angle SNB of 2°, although the intermediate reduction in ANB of 1° seems to be due to a reduction in SNA of that amount.

The strong impression remains that the improvements that are to be seen in the occlusion are not due to changes in the basic face shape but to changes in the arrangement of the teeth within the facial outlines. During the course of treatment the lower incisors have become proclined from 72·5° to the mandibular plane to 92·5°, a change of 20°, and the upper incisors have been retroclined by 6° to the maxillary plane. The changes in the molar region

2. *G. J.* (*Figs.* 188–190).

DIAGNOSIS.—This patient, a boy aged 8 years 8 months, attended showing a severe degree of postnormality of dental bases and a similar discrepancy in the occlusion aggravated by early loss of deciduous teeth and closure of spaces for the unerupted premolar teeth. In this case there was no recorded anomaly of function of the orofacial musculature apart from a posture of the lower lip below the upper incisors. It was envisaged from the outset that teeth should be removed as part of treatment eventually to deal with the problem of crowding. (*Fig.* 188.)

TREATMENT.—A Fränkel 1 appliance was used in view of the severity of the overjet and overbite in an attempt to produce some improvement pending the eruption of the permanent canine and premolar teeth.

Changes for the better began to take place within a few weeks and by the time eight months had passed there was a very marked improvement. (*Fig.* 189). The appliance was worn for a further year because improvement appeared to be continuing. The premolars were then

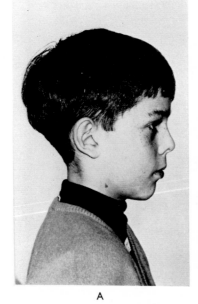
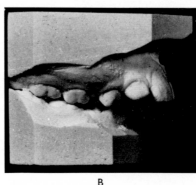
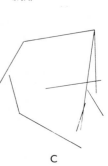

Fig. 188.—G. J., aged 8 years 11 months. A, Profile. B, Models, right lateral view. C, Tracing of X-ray.

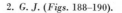

Fig. 189.—G. J., A, Tracing at age 9 years 7 months. B, Tracing at 8 years 11 months and 9 years 7 months superimposed. Upper incisors are retroclined, lower incisors are proclined.

have been noticeable but by no means as striking. The patient's ability to keep a normal lip position and activity has been greatly improved and will be an important factor in the ultimate stability of the new occlusal relationship.

beginning to erupt and after a further six months extraction of the upper first premolars was advised to allow the canine teeth to erupt. (*Fig.* 190).

ASSESSMENT.—What were the changes that took place in this case? There is no doubt of the improvement that occurred in the incisor relationship and the tracings of the cephalometric films seem to show that the change is due to alteration in axial inclinations. It is impossible to say about which point the teeth inclined because the bone areas in which the teeth are supported have changed in position. It should, however, be noted that the relative positions of the anterior part of the jaws themselves as indicated by SNA and SNB remained the same.

The relationship of the molar teeth on the two sides did not behave in the same way. On the right there was little if any change, while on the left a postnormal molar relationship of one unit improved to a half-unit postnormality. There was no obvious explanation as to how this had come about.

PROGNOSIS.—It was noted in this case that there was no anomaly of function apart from a resting of the lower lip below the upper incisors—a condition which no longer obtains as the new incisor relationship now permits correct lip posture at rest. In these circumstances conditions are favourable for stability of the new incisor relationship. The crowding of the dental arches is to be treated by removal of first premolars and the final occlusal relationship of the buccal segments has yet to be worked out.

3. *W. McK.* (*Figs.* 191, 192).

DIAGNOSIS.—This boy, aged 3 years, was brought for advice because of an open bite condition and marked retrognathism. On examination the patient was found to have a postnormal dental base relation, incompetent lips, and a marked lower lip-sucking/tongue-thrusting oral activity. The occlusion was markedly postnormal and

stability. After a total period of twelve months the appliance was withdrawn and the second cephalometric film was taken two months later. (*Fig.* 194.)

An examination of the dental casts and the cephalometric tracings showed that the changes that had taken place were due to a repositioning of the mandible distally and to a slight proclination of the upper incisor teeth.

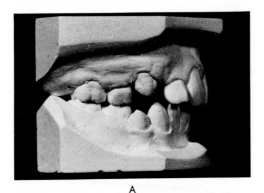

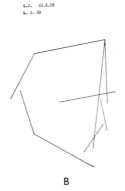

G.J. 22.6.58
4. 1. 69

A B

Fig. 190.—G. J., A, Models at age 10 years 7 months. B, Tracing at 10 years 7 months.

there was a considerable overbite. There was no thumb sucking. (*Fig.* 191.)

TREATMENT.—The patient was given a F.R.1 appliance and took to it at once and has worn the appliance without any difficulty for a year and three months.

There was considerable improvement in the occlusion in that time and the patient is to continue to wear the appliance as long as improvements continue to take place. (*Fig.* 192.) The author is not sure that it would be wise simply to continue to use the appliance indefinitely and if a static condition is reached a resting period from treatment should be allowed, in all probability during the eruption of the permanent dentition, and when these teeth are erupted the whole problem should be reviewed in the light of the circumstances then found.

Prenormal Occlusion

T. K. (*Figs.* 193, 194).

DIAGNOSIS.—This patient, aged 9 years, had a severe Class III malocclusion due in part to a mesial displacement of the mandible on closing from the position of rest to the centric occlusal position, and also to a basic discrepancy in facial proportions in the direction of a mandibular prognathism. The large degree of overlap of the incisors and the break up of the occlusal line in the buccal segments suggest that there is some overclosure in this case, a condition that goes with premature contact, muscle spasm, failure of eruption of teeth in the buccal segments, and reduction of the normal maxillo-mandibular vertical height dimension. (*Fig.* 193.)

TREATMENT.—The condition was treated with a F.R.3 appliance and after a period of four months from the time the appliance was fitted a great improvement in the occlusion had taken place; so much so that correct incisor relationship had been produced. The appliance was worn for a further eight months because the degree of overbite of the incisors was not judged to be sufficient to ensure

The maxillo-mandibular separation also appears to have increased considerably, although the angular position of the mandibular body has not appreciably changed.

A second case of prenormal occlusion was also treated with the F.R.3 appliance and it is interesting to note that there were strong similarities in the general appearance of the occlusion and also in the reaction to treatment. It seemed that in both cases there was an element of displacement so that it is impossible to say from the evidence of these cases what is the effect of the appliance on true Class III malocclusion, that is to say, mandibular prognathism uncomplicated by any mesial displacement.

Open Bite

M. B. (*Figs.* 195, 196).

DIAGNOSIS.—This boy was brought for advice at the age of 6 years with a marked open bite, a tongue thrust, and lip contraction on swallowing and speech. (*Fig.* 195.)

It was felt that little could be accomplished by any form of active treatment in this case and the patient was dismissed for a period of three years, returning at the age of 9 years and 3 months. (*Fig.* 196.)

The permanent incisors had erupted but the open bite condition remained much as it had been when the patient first attended. The patient was dismissed for a further year after which, at the age of 10 years and 3 months, a F.R.1 appliance was fitted and worn for a period of 11 months. During this time a considerable improvement in the open bite condition occurred, after which the appliance was left out. (*Fig.* 197.)

A record of this patient taken seven months later showed no further change in the overbite relationship. It appeared reasonable to conclude that it is very likely that the improvement in the overbite relationship was caused by the use of the appliance rather than that the change was taking place naturally during the time the appliance was being worn.

129

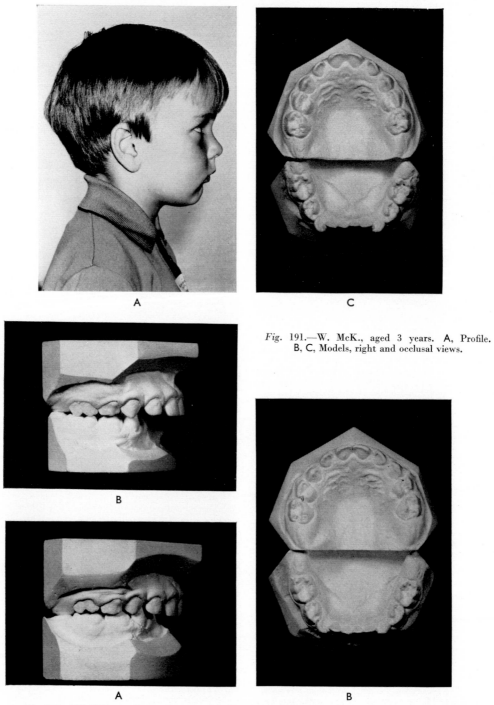

A

C

Fig. 191.—W. McK., aged 3 years. **A**, Profile. **B, C**, Models, right and occlusal views.

B

A

B

Fig. 192.—W. McK., aged 4 years 3 months. **A**, Models, right view. **B**, Occlusal view. Note slight improvement in arrangement of lower incisors.

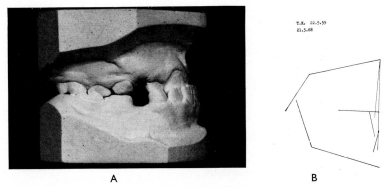

T.K. 22.5.59
21.5.68

A   B

Fig. 193.—T. K., aged 9 years. **A**, Models, right view. **B**, Tracing.

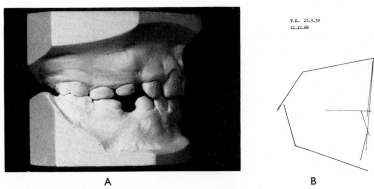

T.K. 22.5.59
12.12.68

A   B

Fig. 194.—T. K., aged 9 years 7 months. **A**, Models, right view. **B**, Tracing.

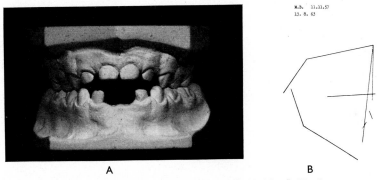

M.B. 11.11.57
13. 8. 63

A   B

Fig. 195.—M. B., aged 5 years 9 months. **A**, Models. **B**, Tracing.

It is interesting to note that during the time when the appliance was being worn there has been, apparently, a forward and upward developmental change in the outline of the mandible. It is tempting to conclude that this must account for the improvement in the overbite. A study of the final stage of seven months over which records were taken shows that the change in mandibular positioning has continued, although the incisor relationship has not continued to improve.

The Remaining Successful Cases.—The other cases in which good results were obtained showed many of the features which have been described in these four subjects. A degree of open bite was often present, possibly due to tongue and lip activities, occlusal relationship

131

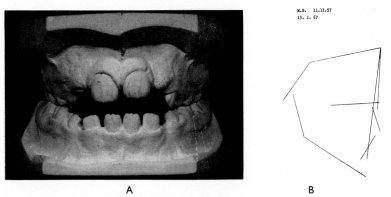

Fig. 196.—M. B., aged 9 years 3 months. A, Models. B, Tracing.

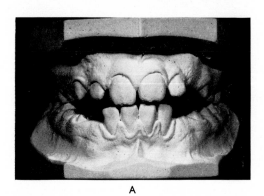

A

Fig. 197.—M. B., aged 11 years. A, Models. B, Tracing. C, Superimposed tracings at 9 years 3 months and 11 years. D, Superimposed tracings at 11 years and 11 years 7 months.

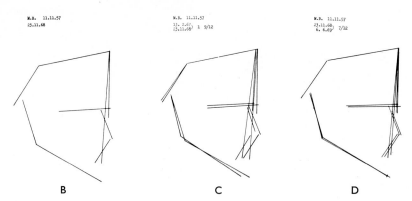

B   C   D

markedly disturbed mesially or distally, and discrepancies in incisor relationships usually severe—postnormally or prenormally. In all the cases that have been examined the changes that have been found to take place appeared to be limited to the dento-alveolar structures. In no case could it be said there was any evidence to suggest that basic jaw relationship had changed in any marked degree. This is surprising in view of the large changes in occlusal relationships, especially in the incisor region, that were observed clinically. Closer examination by means of cephalometric films only revealed changes in tooth inclinations.

132

Changes in skull base angle and in mandibular posture within the craniofacial complex were found but these changes were not reflected in any change in the measurements by which relationship between upper and lower dental bases is usually judged. These observations support the idea that the Fränkel appliance acts by mediating the apposition of bone on surfaces rather than by promoting change in the relationship of the two parts of the masticatory face as a whole. It has been the author's experience that changes in occlusal relationship in the buccal segments mesio-distally do not occur readily or markedly with the F.R.1 appliance, although other authors no doubt have evidence to the contrary.

The Cases that Failed.—And what can be said about the cases that did not improve with the use of the Function Corrector?

The first thing is that in the material available for this investigation the cases that failed were all in the Class II, division 1 group. The subjects did not differ greatly from those in whom the treatment was a success, with one important exception, and this is the group 3 subjects in whom there was a thumb-sucking habit. To some extent it appeared that the influence of the thumb did not counteract the effect of the appliance as such, but rather because the appliance interfered with the activity of the thumb, which was one of the aims of treatment, in the cases in question it was not the thumb which gave way but the appliance.

In one case in which the parent was more than usually active and interested in the progress of treatment it was stated that the appliance was felt to be an affront to the thumb-sucking activity and the thumb was greatly preferred to the appliance. In the other thumb-sucking cases no effect was produced by the appliance at all and, although the day-to-day use of the appliance was not reported and documented, it seemed very likely that the appliances were not worn.

As regards the other four categories these may be divided into those in whom there was non-cooperation in wearing the appliance, although the malocclusions seemed basically amenable to treatment by the system, and

those in whom there was cooperation. In the first of these groups of cases appliances were left out, lost, and broken so that the time during which the appliances were in position must have been very small. It seemed clear that in some of these cases the fault did not lie entirely with the patient. It was found that the appliance was sometimes not comfortable to wear because it was unstable and the screens did not, in consequence, lie in the proper positions or stood too far out from the alveolar process or the tooth crowns. Sometimes the mandible had been brought too far forward, so producing discomfort and difficulty in speech and causing the appliance to tilt and hold the lips in a completely wrong position.

In the remaining cases, as far as could be ascertained, there was good cooperation and parental interest and anxiety to have a good result.

Even so, the results were disappointing, with small changes only or no change at all after wearing the appliances. Two further aspects of these cases in which there was cooperation appeared to be of significance, one of which was that there was a well defined dental base discrepancy and usually associated with this was the fact that there was no anomaly of tongue or lip activity.

CONCLUSIONS

It may be worth while to consider: (1) What should the Fränkel appliance be used for? (2) In what kind of cases may success be hoped for? (3) What is one entitled to expect from the appliance if properly used?

1. The Fränkel appliance has been shown to produce improvement of the occlusion in Class II and Class III malocclusions and in open bite so that any cases of these types may be considered for treatment by the Function Corrector. It has not been the author's experience that the appliance helps the condition of crowding as such, although in some of the successfully treated Class II, division 1 cases crowding was present. The need to extract teeth for the relief of crowding remained and this need was foreseen, although the malocclusion as a whole improved. So far,

133

treatment of Class II, division 2 cases has not been attempted by the present author.

2. The appliance has been found to work successfully in cases in which there is a severe discrepancy of dental base and occlusal relationship; in which there is a severe anomaly of function of the tongue and lips; and in which there has been crowding and early loss of deciduous teeth. In cases in the present series in which there was a thumb-sucking habit no improvement was produced. This may be an indication for caution in the use of the appliance in such cases.

3. What may one expect from the use of the appliance?

a. It is the author's experience that, if the appliance is going to work, changes will take place rapidly. If this does not occur it is likely that the appliance is not going to be successful and after a period of about four months the diagnosis and treatment plan should be carefully reconsidered.

b. The changes that take place are mainly to be seen in the anterior teeth and are produced by changes in axial inclination of the teeth.

c. Changes in the anteroposterior occlusion of the teeth in the buccal segments will be small and it is the author's practice to produce such changes by other means than the Function Corrector.

d. Changes in the relationship of the teeth appear to be produced by rearrangement of the dento-alveolar structures and not by changes in the basal relationships of the jaws.

e. The appliance seems to have a valuable part to play in certain cases in the mixed dentition stage of development when the fitting of precisely constructed removable or fixed appliances may be disturbed by the loss of deciduous teeth.

f. The appliance can be used in young subjects and, when severe malocclusions are present, a start can be given to improvement of occlusal relationship.

g. The relationship between the orthodontist and the patient is important in eliciting co-operation. If the patient does not accept the appliance and virtually forget that it is being worn, treatment by this means will almost certainly fail.

The Function Corrector is a most useful appliance in the treatment of a proportion of cases of certain types. The number of cases included in the present investigation is very small—so small as to make it perhaps unwise to try to draw any general conclusions from them. A careful, accurate, and dispassionate appraisal of the effects of treatment in even a small number of cases can be shown to be informative, revealing, and helpful in the planning of future applications of the system.

THE ORAL SCREEN

The oral screen takes its place among the functional appliances by virtue of the fact that it embodies no active elements designed to produce forces acting on the teeth but produces its effects by controlling or redirecting the pressures which originate in the muscular and soft-tissue curtain of the cheeks and lips.

The oral screen is also used at times to counteract deficiencies in lip posture and function by providing a covering for the anterior teeth and their adjoining gingival tissues and to prevent oral respiration when anterior and posterior oral seals are inadequate.

The value of the oral screen in producing improvements in tooth arrangement and occlusal relationship, in training the labial musculature to improvement in posture and function, in improving the health of the pharyngeal tissues by preventing oral respiration, and through all these means promoting the greater well-being of the patient has for long been a matter of debate. The evidence for the more remote effects and wider implications of treatment with the oral screen has been largely subjective, difficult to record precisely and to distinguish among the changes which could be attributed to growth, development, and variations in the health of patients treated with this appliance.

It is in the region of the lips and labial segments of the dental arches that the oral screen can be used to produce predictable treatment results, and here the effects which the oral screen produces can be recorded with some accuracy and objectivity.

If the upper incisors are proclined and spaced and there is an increase in overjet and the oral incisal edges (*Figs.* 198, 199). If the lower incisors are in contact with the upper incisors in the position of centric occlusion, pressure of the oral screen will be transmitted also to

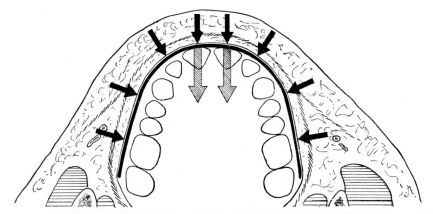

Fig. 198.—The oral screen. The entire pressure of the soft tissues of the lips and cheeks is concentrated on the central incisors. The lateral pressure of the cheeks on the smooth sloping surface of the screen is resolved in a posterior direction. The appliance may be designed to act upon the lateral incisors as well.

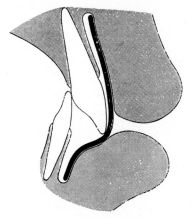

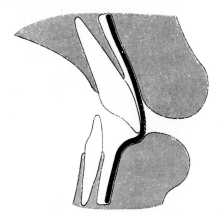

Fig. 199.—An oral screen fitted in a case in which there is proclination of the upper incisor and the lower incisor touches the upper incisors when the teeth are in centric occlusion. In this position the pressure on the upper incisor is also transmitted to the lower incisors. It is doubtful whether the upper incisors can be retroclined in this way.

Fig. 200.—An oral screen fitted in a case in which the upper incisors are proclined and spaced but the lower incisors do not touch the upper incisors when the teeth are in centric occlusion. In these circumstances the oral screen will retrocline the upper incisors.

screen is made so that it touches only the proclined incisors and is not in contact with the teeth in the buccal segments, the pressure of the lips and of the cheeks which lie in contact with the smooth divergent lateral wings of the oral screen will all be concentrated on the labial surfaces of the proclined incisors near the the lower incisors when the teeth are brought together as in swallowing, and this contact of the upper incisors with the lowers will prevent retroclination of the upper incisors.

The use of an oral screen in circumstances such as these is not without risk to the upper incisor teeth themselves, which are pressed

135

from in front by the oral screen and intermittently tapped from behind by the lower incisors at each closure of the teeth into occlusion.

In the course of time resorption of the upper root apices may occur.

If, when the posterior teeth are in occlusion, there is no contact between the upper and lower incisors, there will be no obstacle to a lingual movement of the upper incisors (*Fig.* 200). It is in circumstances like these that the

surface as to rock the upper edge forwards out of control of the upper lip. In either event, the screen cannot be tolerated by the patient.

The mechanical action of the oral screen can be seen, therefore, to be mainly in producing a lingual pressure on the upper incisors, and, in consequence, lingual inclination of these teeth if there is no mechanical obstacle to such a movement. The possibility of producing more far-reaching alterations in occlusal

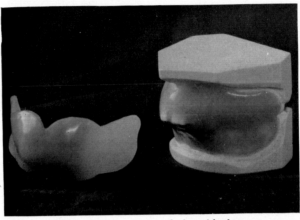

Fig. 201.—The models are fixed in centric occlusion with plaster or wax and covered with a layer of wax labially. Note how the wax curves inwards below the upper incisors. The waxed oral screen is on the left.

upper incisors may be retroclined by means of the oral screen.

In designing an oral screen the relationship of the lower lip to the labial segments of the dental arches is important. In cases in which there is such a degree of overjet that it is only with difficulty that the lower lip can be brought out over the upper incisors, care must be taken to curve the oral screen inwards towards the lower incisors sufficiently to allow the lower lip to slide easily upwards and outwards labially to the oral screen. If, in these circumstances, the screen is brought downwards in a continuous curve over the upper incisors the lower lip may not succeed in reaching out in front of the screen and, lying inside it, may force the screen out of position and expel it from the mouth, or else, reaching out in front of the screen, it may exert such pressure on its labial

relationship, such as reduction in overbite and correction of postnormality of the occlusion, has been suggested from time to time, but the author has not found the oral screen to be effective in these respects.

Construction of the Oral Screen.—The oral screen is constructed on upper and lower working models fixed together in centric occlusion. The impressions from which the models are cast must reproduce the full depth of the labial sulcus.

One thickness of pink modelling wax is applied to the labial aspect of the teeth and the alveolar processes and extended to the limits of the sulcus vertically and distally, allowance being made for the labial and buccal fræna by trimming back the wax as required. This layer of wax is sealed in position and then scraped down over the incisal third of the

136

labial surfaces of the upper incisor teeth which it is desired to retrocline (*Fig.* 201). The thickness of modelling wax is not standardized and if the wax used is not thick enough,

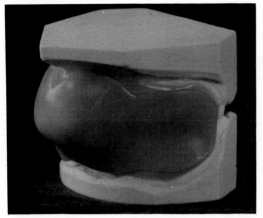

Fig. 202.—The oral screen waxed-up on the models.

additions must be made to the sides of the wax layer in order to leave sufficient clearance between the oral screen and the teeth and alveolar tissues in the buccal region.

Attention must also be paid to the contour of the wax between the incisal edges of the upper incisor and the lower labial sulcus to ensure that the correct curve is provided to accept the lower lip.

The oral screen is then constructed in a single thickness of wax over the surface provided on the working models. The edges of the wax model of the oral screen are taken a little within the limits of the buccal vestibule and allowance is again made for the labial and buccal fræna (*Fig.* 202). The wax of the oral screen can be thickened as may seem necessary to make the final appliance strong enough.

The screen is then thoroughly chilled and invested, outer aspect downwards, in thin cold plaster. As a precaution against warpage during investment, the screen, while still on the model, may be coated with a layer of plaster. When the plaster has set, the coated screen is removed and invested in the deep part of the flask (*Fig.* 203). The second half of the flask is poured into the inside of the screen. The

appliance is finished in clear acrylic resin and smoothed and polished.

If the oral screen is being used to retrocline the upper incisor teeth, additions of clear,

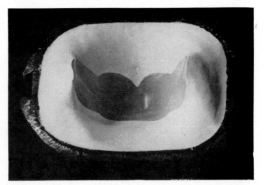

Fig. 203.—The oral screen encased in the flask before casting the top half.

cold-curing, acrylic material may be made to the inside of the appliance as tooth movement takes place, to maintain pressure on the anterior teeth.

The effect of the oral screen in retroclining the upper incisors is shown in *Fig.* 204.

CASE REPORT

M. O'N., aged 8½ years

DIAGNOSIS.—Dental base relation normal, lips competent. Swallows with teeth together. Upper arch well formed, but incisors were proclined and spaced. In the lower arch $\overline{E|}$ had been removed and $\overline{6|}$ had come forwards and closed part of the space for $\overline{5|}$. The overjet was 8–10 mm. and the overbite was incomplete. The patient sucked her thumb.

TREATMENT.—An oral screen was worn for one year, at the end of which time the upper incisors were retroclined into contact with the lower incisors and the patient had ceased the thumb-sucking habit.

THE LOWER INCLINED PLANE

The lower inclined plane is an appliance used for the treatment of an incorrect biting relationship of the upper and lower incisors, that is to say when one or a number of upper incisors bite lingually to the lower incisors. The appliance consists of a polished metal or acrylic resin plane inclined at about 45° to the occlusal plane and placed between the upper and lower incisors in such a way that the upper incisor or incisors bite on the plane and are

137

guided into their correct position labially to the lower incisors. (*Fig.* 205.)

Indications and Contra-indications for the Use of the Lower Inclined Plane.—The lower inclined plane is useful when the incisor teeth are at a relatively early stage of eruption and where there is a good degree of overbite. In used. It may be impossible to produce the necessary degree of upper incisor proclination and if the overbite becomes reduced at all it may be impossible to produce correct incisor relationship in the end.

Design and Construction of the Lower Inclined Plane.—The most satisfactory inclined plane

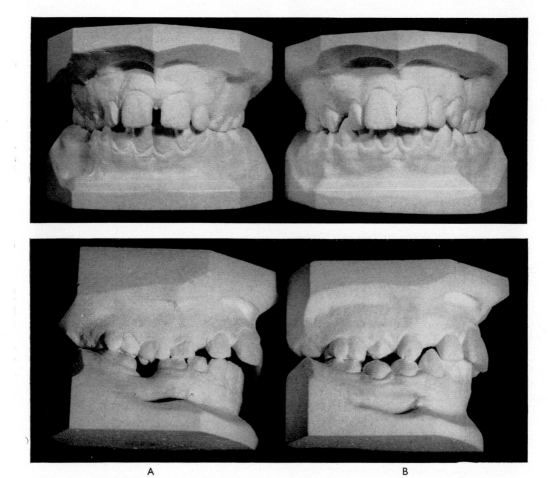

A   B

Fig. 204.—Treatment with the oral screen. A, Before treatment—the upper incisors are proclined and spaced, but there is no obstacle to their retroclination; B, After treatment.

cases where many deciduous teeth have been removed, rendering the temporary propping open of the bite difficult, the inclined plane is useful. (*Figs.* 206, 207.)

If there is a marked degree of mandibular prognathism and the overbite of the incisors is not great the inclined plane should not be is the removable, clear acrylic plane. Sometimes cemented inclined planes and planes in a cast metal such as silver are recommended, but both have great drawbacks. If a plane is cemented, it is impossible to check progress in the tooth movement unless the appliance is removed, and this may entail cutting or

138

damaging the plane. Cast metal planes are hardly worth the additional time and expense of construction.

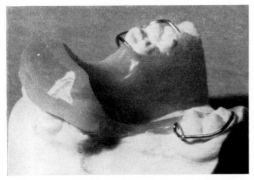

Fig. 205.—A lower removable inclined plane clasped on 6|6. If there are no back teeth the buccal gum pads should be covered with extensions of the baseplate.

A removable acrylic plane is made on a stone model from an alginate impression. A good coating of separating material is painted on to the model.

Two clasps should be placed at the posterior ends of the baseplate if there are suitable teeth present. If all the lower back teeth have been removed, as occasionally happens, the baseplate should be thickened a little and carried over the occlusal surface of the gum pads. The resulting flanges help the patient in retaining the appliance.

The inclined plane is built up, slightly capping the incisor and canine teeth, and the appliance is finished in clear acrylic material.

When fitting the appliance any undercuts in the resin due to tilted or imbricated teeth should be carefully eased away with fine

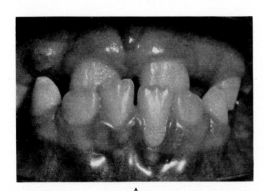
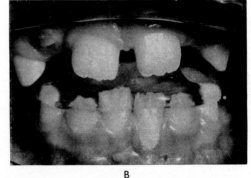

| A | B |

Fig. 206.—A, Lingual occlusion of 1|1 which are recently erupted. B, The inclined plane in position with the upper incisors biting on it.

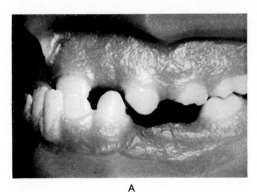
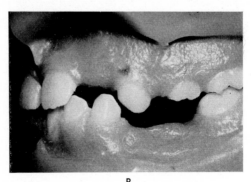

| A | B |

Fig. 207.—Photographs of acrylic models of the treatment of the patient shown in Fig. 206. A, Before treatment. B, After treatment.

stones and fissure burs until the appliance goes in easily but positively.

The inclined plane is finally adjusted for height and angulation by grinding the slope against a 3-in. rotating lathe wheel. The plane is finally polished.

The appliance should be worn full time and the patient instructed to cut up food and adopt a soft diet until the incisor relationship is correct and the appliance can be removed.

Treatment should only take a matter of weeks and if improvement does not appear to be taking place soon, a thorough check should be made on the wearing of the appliance and the diagnosis of the case.

CHAPTER XII

ROTATION AND ROOT MOVEMENT OF TEETH

REMOVABLE appliances are not on the whole as efficient as fixed appliances for rotation and root movement of teeth, and it is important, therefore, to exercise discretion in attempting these movements with removable appliances. There are, however, certain rotation and root

may be applied, and this requirement automatically eliminates the possibility of rotating certain teeth. For instance, canines, upper and lower, are of a rounded shape which does not offer two points near the outside of the contour of the tooth to which suitable pressures may

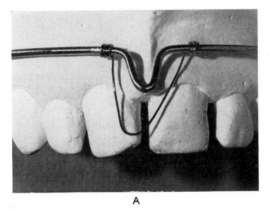
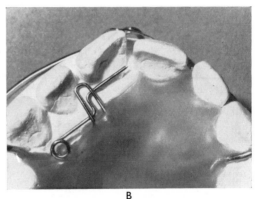

A   B

Fig. 208.—**A**, This cantilever spring (0·3 mm. thick), attached to the arch by soldering, impinges only on the mesial edge of the tooth. The wide curve of the spring gives stability mesiodistally. **B**, The lingual spring (0·5 mm. thick) impinges on the distal edge of the tooth, so completing the *couple*.

movements that removable appliances can perform very well and it is helpful to bear these possibilities in mind when considering treatment problems.

The production of a rotary movement requires the application of two equal and opposite pressures acting at a distance apart to produce a *mechanical couple*.★ This will produce rotation about a point somewhere between the lines of action of the two forces. It is therefore necessary to find, on a tooth to be rotated, two points at a suitable distance apart on which pressures in opposite directions

─────────────────

★ " A couple consists of two equal parallel forces which act in opposite directions. When acting on a rigid body, it cannot produce motion in any particular direction since the algebraic sum of its resolved parts in that direction is zero; it follows that its effect is to produce rotation."—Borchardt, W. G., *A School Certificate Mechanics and Hydrostatics.*

be applied. Lower incisors, again, are so small in section that the forces even when applied at the extreme ends of the incisal edge are so close together that an effective mechanical couple cannot be produced.

It is important when constructing appliances for rotation and root movement to ensure that the springs act exactly at the points intended and do not slide away to some other nearby but unsuitable point. For this reason it is sometimes necessary to make springs rather stiff in order to ensure accuracy of application to the teeth and to accept the short range of action inherent in such springs. The straight cantilever spring as used in other situations should be used as far as possible, as this spring can be made to act with the greatest precision on any desired part of a tooth. These springs may, as before, be made of varying thicknesses of wire with various numbers of coils at the point of attachment.

ROTATION OF UPPER INCISORS

This may be done with two cantilever springs pressing at opposite ends of the incisal edge producing the mechanical couple already referred to. In the example shown, *Fig.* 208 A, B, on the outer edge of the tooth. The labial spring is made in a wide curve so as to be as stable as possible in a mesiodistal direction and so that slight accidental alteration in its mesiodistal position will not affect the point of application of the spring. It is thus possible to secure precision in the point of application of the pressure with a long range of action,

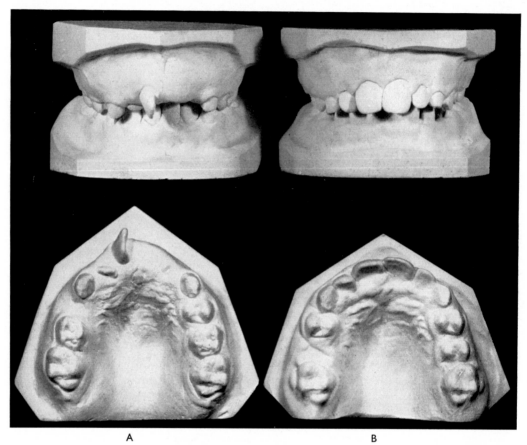

A   B

Fig. 209.—Rotation of 1| by means of a removable appliance. A, 1| has erupted in a position of rotation of 90°. |1 has failed so far to erupt. B, 1| has been rotated into correct position. Active treatment, 5 months. |1 exposed surgically and erupted into correct position after 4–5 months. Patient aged 9 years.

the two springs differ in range of action but the pressures they exert are the same. It will be seen that these springs are designed to act as near to the outer edge of the tooth as possible. The lingual spring is cranked to increase the efficiency of the guard, and the operating end is bent so as to impinge exactly without making the spring too stiff and rigid. The possibilities for such rotations with removable appliances are shown in *Fig.* 209.

There is not always much room for the placement of a finger spring lingually for the rotation of an incisor and a more compact and rather stronger spring is shown in *Fig.* 210.

142

This is a small apron spring with two transverse torque bars, one at either side. The spring is made of 0·35-mm. hard wire. The labial springs are also of simple design, 0·7-mm. wire with a looped end which makes it easy to put pressure exactly on the distal edge of the

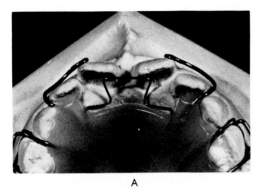

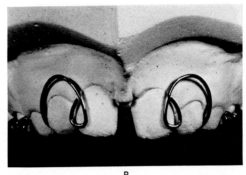

A   B

Fig. 210.—Rotation of incisors. A, The lingual spring consists of an apron with a torque bar at either side. The elasticity of the spring comes mainly from the transverse sections which twist slightly, the apron part of the spring bending hardly at all. B, The labial springs are 0·7-mm. wire with large end loops which cross the distal edges of the teeth and are activated lingually.

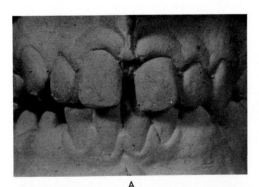

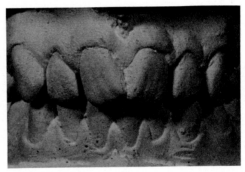

A   B

tooth. Both these types of springs can be used on single teeth, naturally enough, although in the case shown two teeth were corrected simultaneously. (Fig. 211.)

Upper lateral incisors can usually be rotated in the same way as central incisors provided that the crowns are well formed and there is a definite, straight incisal edge.

ROTATION OF CANINES AND LOWER INCISORS

As already mentioned, the rotation of these teeth is not readily performed with removable appliances and is in fact much better performed with fixed appliances.

C

Fig. 211.—Correction of 1|1. A, The frænum was excised and the appliance shown in Fig. 210 fitted. B, 1|1 have been over-rotated. C, One year later, after six months' retention, the central incisors have settled into correct position.

143

ROTATION OF PREMOLARS
AND MOLARS

The rotation of these teeth is not a very frequently required movement, and in many cases in which such rotation is required a fixed appliance will be necessary in order to ensure accuracy of placement of the crown in

biting buccally to the lower first premolar (*Figs.* 212 A, 213 A). Rotation of the upper premolar by swinging the lingual cusp distally will produce correct occlusion (*Figs.* 212 B, 213 B). This rotation may be performed by pressing firmly on the mesial surface of the tooth opposite the lingual cusp. The buccal cusp

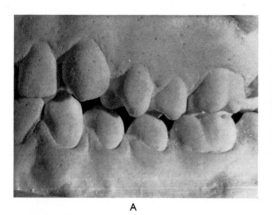 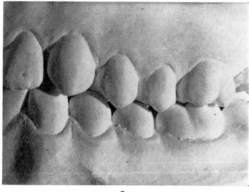

A   B

Fig. 212.—Distal rotation of upper first premolar producing correct occlusal relation with the lower. The condition was bilateral.

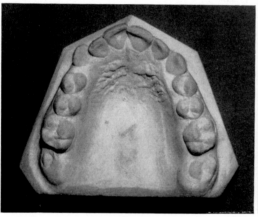 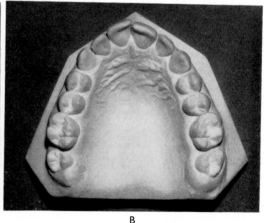

A   B

Fig. 213.—The rotation of upper first premolars distally by means of pressure on the mesiolingual aspect.

its new position and to ensure rotation of the tooth about the desired axis. There are, however, certain situations in which premolars and molars can be rotated with a straightforward removable appliance. A common misplacement of the upper first premolar is to find the lingual cusp rotated mesially and

rests against the mesial surface of the tooth behind and the tooth rotates about its point of contact with the second premolar (*Fig.* 214 A, B). It will be noticed that here only one force is used and that the place of the second is taken by a fixed point, the point of contact, between the first and second premolars. We

144

have, therefore, in this case not strictly a couple but a force rotating about a point. The value of the force for rotation purposes is point is comparatively small, the value of this moment is low, hence the rotating effort is small. It is found clinically that

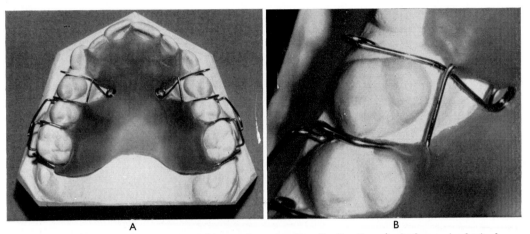

A   B

Fig. 214.—Appliance for rotation of upper first premolars distally. Note **A**, Anchorage is obtained from all the other teeth in the arch except the canines; **B**, The spring is applied with great accuracy to the mesial surface of the tooth opposite the lingual cusp.

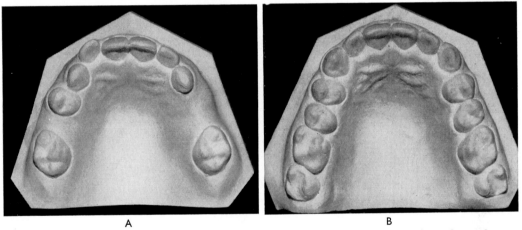

A   B

Fig. 215.—**A**, **B**, Distal rotation of left upper first permanent molar to facilitate eruption of second premolar.

given by the *moment* of the force about this point.* As the distance between the line of action of the force and the

* " The tendency of a force . . . to turn a body round a given point . . . is measured by the product of the magnitude of the force and the length of the perpendicular drawn from the point on its line of action, this product . . . being called the moment of the force about the given point."—Borchardt, W. G., *A School Certificate Mechanics and Hydrostatics*.

rotations such as this take a considerable time.

The rotation of lower premolars in this way is not likely to be very successful as these teeth are usually almost circular in section and the formation of a mechanical couple to rotate them is difficult or impossible.

Another common tooth misplacement is the mesiolingual rotation of the upper first

145

permanent molar, which considerably reduces the space required for the second premolar (*Fig.* 215 **A**). This tooth may be rotated distally by pressure on the mesial surface opposite to the mesiobuccal cusp

ROOT MOVEMENT

This term refers to the tipping of apices deliberately in one direction or the other, a movement that is usually performed with most of the fixed appliances, and there is little, if

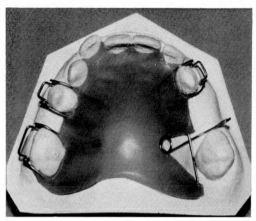

Fig. 216.—Appliance for distal rotation of upper first permanent molar. The spring, of 0·6-mm. wire, presses on the tooth opposite to the mesiobuccal cusp. Rotation takes place about the palatal root.

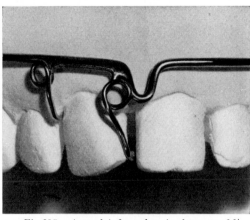

Fig. 217.—A *couple* is formed to tip the apex of 1| mesially. These springs are short and stiff, 0·6 mm. thick, and are applied with great accuracy as far apart as possible on the mesial and distal surfaces of the incisor. The ends of the springs are flattened and turned in to impinge squarely on the tooth.

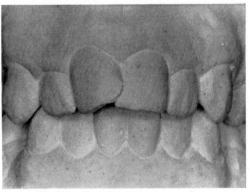

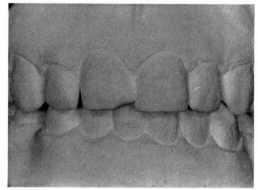

Fig. 218.—Mesial root movement of upper right central incisor. Room was also made for the central incisors by extraction of first premolars.

(*Fig.* 216). Rotation takes place about the palatal root (*Fig.* 215B).

The crowns of lower molars are not of a shape that facilitates rotation by means of pressure on any part of their mesial surfaces and the roots are of a shape and size that are resistant to rotation. These teeth are better rotated when necessary by means of fixed appliances.

any, scope in this particular sphere for the effective use of removable appliances. At the same time if it is desired to tilt the roots of an upper incisor mesially or distally, this may be attempted with a fair prospect of success by applying equal and opposite pressures to the mesial and distal surfaces of the crown of the tooth near the incisal edge and at the cervical margin.

146

The appliance shown in *Fig.* 217 will produce these pressures. The tooth has to be approached from the labial side in order to avoid the bite of the lower incisors and to get a point of application at the gingival margin but this will be no disadvantage in this instance because root movement is usually slow, so that quite long intervals can be allowed between adjustments of the springs (*Fig.* 218).

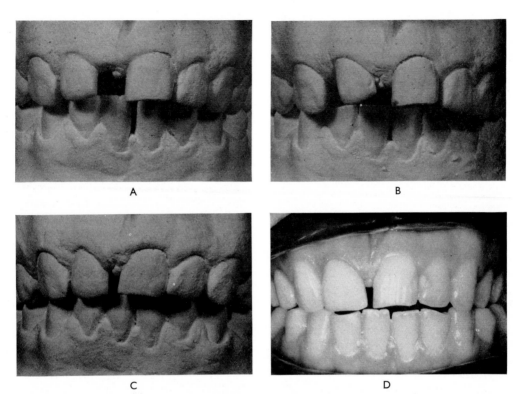

A   B

C   D

Fig. 219.—Root movement of an upper lateral incisor. A, In this case there was postnormal occlusion with increased overjet and 1| had been accidentally damaged and was extracted. B, 2| has been tipped mesially by a palatal finger spring. C, 2| has been uprighted by a mesial pressure near the anatomical neck by means of a palatal finger spring, while a counter pressure was applied in a distal direction near to the incisal edge on the mesial surface of the crown. The incisors have also been retroclined. D, 2| has been crowned and, due to a slight relapse of the retroclined incisors, there is a small space between the crowned lateral incisor and |1.

as nearly as possible in the same plane as the incisal edge. In order to separate the points of application of the pressures as widely as possible the lower spring should be applied as near as possible to the incisal edge and the upper spring may be applied actually below the gum margin by grinding the end of the spring flat and slipping it into the gingival trough. The springs are made of a fairly heavy wire, 0·6 mm., and coiled for resilience. They will, even so, have a short range of action,

Fig. 219 shows another case of root movement of an upper incisor followed by jacket crowning.

Root movement of other teeth in other directions is a haphazard and unreliable procedure with removable appliances and is not as a rule undertaken. The possibility of tipping upper incisor roots labially and lingually is one possibility that is open to exploration, but no results of such attempts are on record up to date.

147

CHAPTER XIII

WELDING FOR ORTHODONTIC APPLIANCE CONSTRUCTION

THE merits of stainless steel as an orthodontic material were recognized many years ago but enthusiasm for the new metal was tempered by the early difficulties that were encountered in producing satisfactory joints in it. The application of resistance welding methods, however, proved a promising approach to the problem and before long welded stainless-steel appliances became firmly established in their own right (Charlier, 1928; De Coster, 1931a, b, 1932).

Spot welding, which is one of the resistance welding processes, is a convenient method for uniting pieces of metal of the same kind. It is also possible to spot weld certain dissimilar metals. The method is clean and quick and produces joints which are strong and reliable; most metals may be spot welded.

The process consists essentially of raising the temperature of the pieces of metal to be joined until the metal becomes plastic but not molten at the site of the proposed joint and immediately applying pressure so that the metal parts are squeezed together in their plastic state and become one. This is strictly comparable to the working of wrought iron by red heat and the hammer on an anvil. Red heat renders the iron plastic; hammering, which is a method of applying powerful pressure, forces the elements of the joint indissolubly into one another's structure.

The resistance welder uses electric current to produce heat in the metal parts which are to be welded. In spot welding the pieces of metal to be united are held together in the required position and placed between two copper or copper alloy rods or electrodes which press the parts together under controlled pressure. In large industrial welders the pressure may be provided by hydraulic, pneumatic, or mechanical means. In small

bench machines spring pressure is usually employed. When current is passed from one electrode to the other through the metal, heat is generated in and between the metal parts which is sufficient to make them plastic. The pressure of the electrodes then forces the metal parts together, so creating the weld.

THE WELDING CIRCUIT

That part of the circuit which is actually used to heat the metal for welding is operated at low voltage, 2–10 volts, and makes use of a high current density. Current is usually provided by the mains alternating current electrical supply using a transformer to step down the voltage to the necessary low level. The transformer is of large capacity so that a heavy current may be passed through the secondary winding; this is important as the heating effect of a current varies as the square of its amperage (I^2) and an adequate current density must be available to perform a resistance weld of any kind.

It is possible to use a heavy-duty storage battery to produce welds (Bell, 1932) but welding equipment based on such a supply usually has to be home-made and the mains-operated welder is to be preferred on grounds of freedom from maintenance problems, reliability, and consistency in welding. Furthermore, a storage battery is limited in the current density it can deliver and it may prove difficult to perform a weld in heavier materials without increasing the time factor to an undesirable degree.

The circuit of a mains-operated welder is shown in *Fig.* 220. The transformer is of substantial construction and the secondary winding is of thick copper wire and has very few turns; in fact only a single turn or loop of copper may be used. The leads from the

148

secondary winding and the electrode holders are similarly heavy in section. The electrodes themselves complete the secondary side of the electrical circuit. These are of copper or more

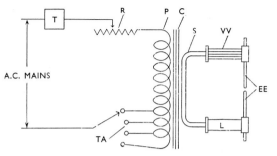

Fig. 220.—The electrical circuit of a spot welder. P, Primary winding of transformer; C, Core of transformer; S, Secondary winding of transformer; T, Timing switch. This may be simple mechanical, automatic mechanical, electrically operated mechanical, or electronic. TA, Tappings on primary winding; R, Variable resistance; VV, Flexible vanes which carry current to upper electrode and also permit vertical movement of the upper electrode. Alternatively a hinging movement of the upper electrode holder may be arranged or this electrode holder may move on a vertical slide. L, Lower electrode holder; this is rigid. EE, Electrodes.

usually of a copper alloy which is harder while having almost the same electrical conductivity.

The primary side of the circuit consists of the primary winding, which is designed to conduct the mains voltage supply of the district in which the equipment is used, and a switch, or timing mechanism, which controls the length of time for which current is permitted to flow. Tappings are usually provided in the primary winding, which make it possible to vary the output of the transformer by varying the voltage in the secondary side of the circuit. In some welders a variable resistance is also provided in series with the primary winding of the transformer to give additional control of the welding heat.

When a weld is made, the workpieces are placed together between the electrodes which exert a controlled pressure on them as already mentioned. The arrangement of electrode—metal part—metal part—electrode makes up a circuit of greatly varying resistance for the current to pass through (*Fig.* 221). The

electrodes, being made of copper alloy, have a very low resistance. The workpieces have usually a higher resistance than the copper electrodes. The sites of contact between the electrodes and the workpieces have again a higher resistance and the resistance in the site of contact between the workpieces themselves is higher still.

When current is passed through this circuit heat is generated in proportion to the electrical resistance of the various parts.★ This means that in the electrodes themselves little heat is

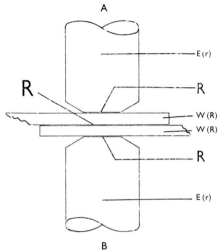

Fig. 221.—Variation in electrical resistance between the electrodes. Between A, in the upper electrode, and B, in the lower electrode, electrical resistance varies greatly. In the electrodes themselves E, E, resistance is small, r. In the workpieces W, W, resistance is usually greater, R. Between the electrodes and the workpieces resistance is greater still R, R. Between the workpieces resistance is greatest, R. Heat produced is directly proportional to the resistance of the part of the circuit through which the current is flowing. The current is the same in every part of the circuit.

developed, while between the workpieces sufficient heat is developed to make the metal plastic and permit a weld to take place (*see Fig.* 222). Heat is also developed between the

★ When current passes through a circuit heat is generated according to the relationship $H = KI^2 RT$, where H = heat in joules, I = current in amperes; R is resistance in ohms; T is time of application of the current in seconds; and K is a constant.

149

electrodes and the workpieces, but this does not produce fusion of the electrodes to the workpieces because copper has a high thermal conductivity, and heat produced at this site is rapidly conducted away. Industrial welders are usually provided with water-cooled electrodes as the machines are designed to make welds at a high rate of repetition.

is generated at the interface of the workpieces. The penetration of softening of the metal should be between one-third to four-fifths of the thickness of the workpieces (Rossi, 1954). The longer the time allowed for a weld, the greater the opportunity for heat developed at the interface to spread into the surrounding metal and the greater the possibility of the

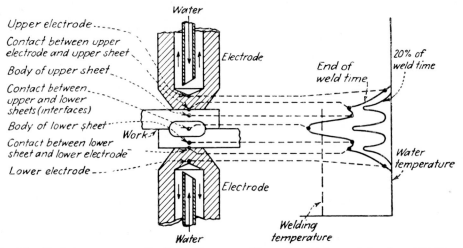

Fig. 222.—Typical temperature distribution in spot welding. (*By kind permission from "Welding Engineering" by E. Rossi. Copyright, 1954, McGraw-Hill Book Co., Inc.*)

ORTHODONTIC WELDER DESIGN

Spot welding is carried out without the aid of flux or any other protecting material so that as the temperature of the workpieces is raised, oxidization and breakdown of the composition of materials which are alloys can occur, which will produce weakness in the weld. These effects can be avoided by various means. It is feasible, for instance, in industrial circumstances to perform spot welds in an inert atmosphere of nitrogen which eliminates oxidization.

It has been found more practical, however, for orthodontic and other purposes making use of fine-gauge wires and sheets of metal, to reduce oxidization and breakdown of metal structure by keeping the time taken to perform welds as short as possible. The shorter the time during which the workpieces are kept at welding temperature, the less oxidization and disturbance of metal structure can take place. The heat required for spot welding

full workpiece thickness rising to a temperature at which loss of temper and softening can occur. Shortening the time allowed for a spot weld, therefore, limits the heating of the workpieces to the interface where heat is required and prevents softening of the full thickness of the metal which would destroy its properties as a spring material. Welding machines for orthodontic and similar materials are, therefore, designed to deliver heavy currents for accurately predetermined, very short times.

Pioneer work on the design of a welder for orthodontic purposes was done by Friel and McKeag (Friel, 1933; Friel and McKeag, 1939), and resulted in the conversion of a small industrial machine into a satisfactory orthodontic welder with a semi-automatic mechanical timing switch.

When using this machine, pressure on a lever or pedal first brings the electrodes together; further pressure on the pedal or

150

lever operates the switch directly. The timing of the weld depends, therefore, on the speed with which the pedal is depressed after the electrodes have been brought into contact. Although the method of timing would seem prone to irregularity, a little practice makes it possible to produce perfectly satisfactory results. One or two of these machines are still in existence.

A second welder has been shown in illustration (Friel and McKeag, 1939) which features upper

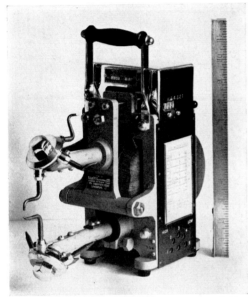

Fig. 223.—The Watkin welder. Features of this welder are the compact size and the electrode design, which facilitate access to confined spaces. The timing switch is automatic mechanical, tappings are provided on the transformer. The upper electrode carrier is hinged. (*By kind permission of Mr. Harold G. Watkin and Elliott and Co. (Liverpool) Ltd.*)

and lower turret electrodes bearing four points each but no details of this machine are given.

The Watkin welder, of portable dimensions, has been widely and successfully used for many years (*Fig. 223*). This machine is fitted with a fully automatic timing switch of mechanical design. Pressure on the foot control first brings the electrodes together; further pressure winds up a spring inside the timing mechanism and when the pedal is fully depressed, the switch mechanism is

released and timing of the weld is thereafter automatically performed.

A timing scale is provided which gives predetermined settings of $\frac{1}{50}$ sec., $\frac{1}{25}$ sec., and four further progressively increasing times.

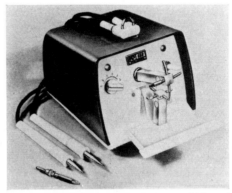

Fig. 224.—The Rocky Mountain 660 Welder. A miniaturized multi-purpose welder. This welder measures $6\frac{3}{4}$ in. high and is designed to spot weld, electro-solder, and heat treat orthodontic wires. (*By kind permission of Rocky Mountain Dental Products Company, Denver, Colorado.*)

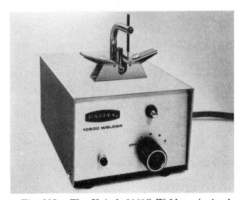

Fig. 225.—The Unitek 1060C Welder. A simple spot welder with plain electrodes. Other models of this manufacture are available with turret electrodes, soldering, and heat treatment accessories. (*By kind permission of the Unitek Corporation, Monrovia, California.*)

Welding is normally carried out at $\frac{1}{25}$ sec. and power is adjusted by selection of a suitable tapping on the transformer. The additional increased timings are provided for use in conjunction with the maximum power on the

151

transformer tapping scale when very heavy gauge materials are to be welded, as, for instance, in plate work.

Small, efficient and very portable bench-top welders are manufactured by the Rocky Mountain Dental Products Company and also by the Unitek Corporation (*Figs.* 224, 225).

The timing of alternating current for very short periods, that is, less than a few cycles or about $\frac{1}{10}$ sec., presents certain problems. Recent developments in electronic engineering, however, have led to the production of equipment for the accurate measurement of very short intervals of time. An electronically timed welder of the half-cycle type operates on a time scale from zero up to a maximum of $\frac{1}{100}$ sec., which means that the maximum time that it will allow for a weld is $\frac{1}{100}$ sec. Welds are normally performed at about $\frac{1}{200}$ sec., more or less, and it is possible to weld materials substantially thicker than those used in orthodontic work on such a machine (*Fig.* 226). The electronic welder makes use of the characteristics of alternating current itself to effect timing. The chief advantage of such a machine is the great accuracy of timing and consistency in welding that it achieves.

The size of the transformer and timing equipment is such that the electronic welder just described must be built into a bench or mobile table permanently. There is, however, now available a portable, bench-top electronically controlled welder of the same manufacture.

A further and interesting type of welding machine which eliminates the need for special switching gear is the capacitor welder (Parfitt and Friel, 1946). A capacitor is charged to a high voltage and when discharged through a transformer the discharge takes place completely in a fraction of a second, so achieving rapid, automatic timing. Several practical problems arise with this type of welder. First, the primary side of the circuit may have to operate at a high voltage, which creates difficulties in the production of a machine for routine workshop or surgery use; secondly, the capacitor required for such a machine is large and bulky and usually takes several seconds to charge up, which may cause an irritating delay between welds.

Some small modern bench-top welders which work on the capacitor principle are now available, but owing to the low voltages and capacitances used power output may sometimes be found to be insufficient for thicker wires.

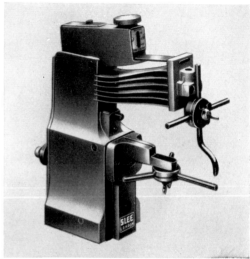

Fig. 226.—The welding head of an electronic welder. The control unit of this welder provides timing control from 0 to 1/100 sec. and voltage control by means of tappings on the transformer. A variable resistance is fitted in series with the primary winding. Electrode pressure may also be varied. The flexible vane system carrying the upper electrode carrier provides vertical movement of the upper electrode with elimination of troubles arising from wear in joints or slides and consequent lateral shake in the upper electrode. The welding head measures $6\frac{3}{4}$ in. high overall. (*By kind permission of the South London Electrical Equipment Co. Ltd.*)

Electrode Design.—Electrode design is an important feature in orthodontic welders. Usually a variety of fine, specially shaped electrode tips are required for the welding of wires, latches, and attachments in fixed appliance construction. Furthermore, certain construction methods demand the welding of appliances which are on plaster models, so making access difficult, which sometimes leads to the production of long and spindly electrodes to facilitate reaching into awkward corners.

Both these special requirements of fineness of electrode tips and length and slenderness for ease of access conflict with the basic welding principles that electrodes should be short and

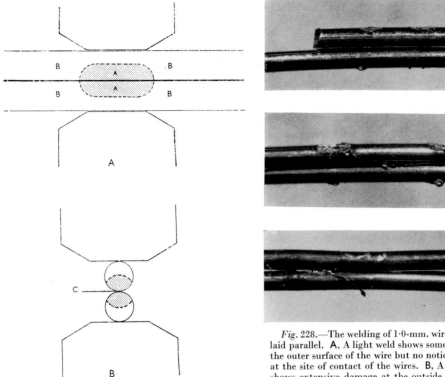

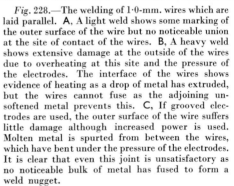

Fig. 228.—The welding of 1·0-mm. wires which are laid parallel. **A**, A light weld shows some marking of the outer surface of the wire but no noticeable union at the site of contact of the wires. **B**, A heavy weld shows extensive damage at the outside of the wires due to overheating at this site and the pressure of the electrodes. The interface of the wires shows evidence of heating as a drop of metal has extruded, but the wires cannot fuse as the adjoining un-softened metal prevents this. **C**, If grooved elec-trodes are used, the outer surface of the wire suffers little damage although increased power is used. Molten metal is spurted from between the wires, which have bent under the pressure of the electrodes. It is clear that even this joint is unsatisfactory as no noticeable bulk of metal has fused to form a weld nugget.

Fig. 227.—The welding of wires. **A**, If the wires are laid parallel, and flat electrodes are used, heating occurs in the area **A**, **A**. Softening should not penetrate more than four-fifths of the thickness of the wires. Support at **B, B, B, B** of unsoftened wire prevents fusion of softened areas into a weld nugget. **B**, Cross-section of the resulting weld shows how very little fusion of metal can take place in such circumstances.

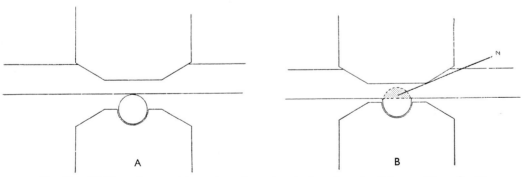

Fig. 229.—Welding wires at right angles using grooved electrodes. **A**, Before welding; **B**, After welding. Note how the groove protects the outer surface of the wire and how all heating and fusion take place at the point of contact of the wires which sink into one another forming a weld nugget, **N**.

153

bulky so that they will conduct electricity to the weld, and heat away from it, with the greatest efficiency. As in most things, compromise is necessary and experience shows that an occasional liberty may be taken in electrode shaping when necessity is urgent.

Most orthodontic welders are provided with a variety of upper and lower electrodes set on rotating turrets so that any pair of upper and lower may be selected at will. A well-designed set of turret electrodes will combine the optimum in ease of access to awkward corners in a plaster model bearing a fixed appliance and conformity with the desirability of shortness and thickness in the electrodes. When filing the tips of electrodes to fit into angles and corners of special attachments, reduction of the bulk of the electrode tip unnecessarily should be avoided.

WELDING FOR APPLIANCE CONSTRUCTION

The material usually employed for appliance construction is 18/8 stainless steel alloy. This metal can be spot welded quite easily; the main difficulties that occur arise either in connexion with the welding of pieces of dissimilar bulk, or with the welding of wires. Flat materials do not present any great problem provided welds are not overheated and the structure of the metal damaged and thereby weakened. Welds made in such materials only occupy small spots surrounded by comparatively large areas of unaffected metal, so that such welds have great strength.

Electrodes for welding tapes should have flat smooth ends and should have adequate bulk to permit free flow of current and to conduct heat away from the weld. The area of the tips of the electrodes should be adequate, about 1–2 mm. across being usually suitable. Sharply pointed electrodes should be avoided as liable to produce burning and pitting of the weld owing to the high resistance of the contact area with the workpiece and consequent overheating. Electrodes of too large an end section may, paradoxically enough, also produce similar defects in welding, as not all of the end surface may be pressed evenly in contact with the metal, especially in a small

bench-type of machine. Irregularities in adaptation of this kind may lead to burns and pits in welding flat materials.

Hard stainless-steel wires as used for orthodontic appliances should, wherever possible, be welded at right angles to one another using grooved electrodes. Joints made in this way are stronger than those made with wires laid parallel to one another.

If wires are laid parallel to one another and flat electrodes used to make the weld, the stiffness of the wire on either side of the weld prevents the forging together of the heated metal (*Figs.* 227, 228 A). If the welding power is increased in an attempt to heat the metal sufficiently to permit forging of the weld, it is found that damage is inflicted on the outer surface of the wire, but the surfaces in contact still do not collapse and form a "weld nugget".★ The support of the unsoftened wire on either side of the weld prevents forging together from taking place (*Fig.* 228 B).

It is interesting to note in *Fig.* 228 C that if grooved electrodes are used to weld wires laid parallel, welding power can be substantially increased without causing damage to the outer contour of the wire. The wire is now heated right through and the upper wire has bent under the pressure of the electrodes as the two wires are forced together, but even under these circumstances no noticeable fusion of the two wires has taken place, no weld nugget has formed. The stiff unsoftened wire on either side of the weld has prevented any useful compression of the weld itself.

If, however, the electrodes are grooved and the wires are laid at right angles (*Figs.* 229, 230) when the weld is made the two wires can be forged together without any distortion of their outer contours. This is because the hollow of the electrode spreads the current over a large surface area so reducing the heating effect at the surface of the wire. The current is concentrated at the contact points of the wires and here the maximum heating effect occurs. The outer contours of the wires have not been

---

★ *Nugget*: The metal joining the parts in spot, seam, or projection welds (Rossi, 1954).

damaged or the metal softened at this situation; this contributes greatly to the strength of the joint and retains the essential properties of the wires for arch or spring purposes. A joint of this

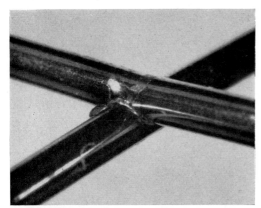

Fig. 230.—1·0-mm. wires welded at right angles, using grooved electrodes. Note the fusion of the wires and the preservation of their outer contour.

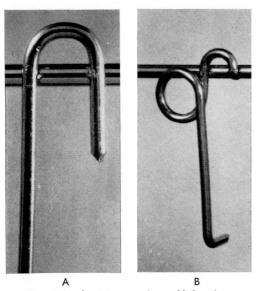

A   B

Fig. 231.—**A**, 0·7-mm. wire welded twice to 1·0-mm. arch. **B**, An auxiliary spring constructed by welding 0·7-mm. wire to 1·0-mm. labial bow.

kind represents the strongest single weld between two wires. If further strength is sought it is possible to weld wires at two points by turning one of them in a small half-circle and in this way a joint of double strength can be made. It is usually feasible, with a little

care, to incorporate such a loop in most situations without inconvenience (*Fig.* 231).

Much of the difficulty of welding spring wires appears to arise from the fact that they are hard; soft stainless steel orthodontic wires can be spot welded very easily and strongly with grooved electrodes.

HEAT BALANCE

Problems arise to some extent in welding light parts to heavy parts in that the heavy parts require more heat to raise them to welding temperature than do light parts and there is a tendency to overheat the light part in the effort to get the heavy part up to the necessary degree of heat.

The problem is largely solved by the fact that heat is developed at the point of contact of the two workpieces, that is exactly at the site of the proposed joint, and if the weld is made quickly enough it is completed before the heat is conducted away into the bulk of the heavy part. In other words, when welding a light part to a heavy part the bulk of the heavy part is not raised to welding temperature, but only a skin at the surface making contact with the light part becomes plastic.

In practice, light tapes can be welded to heavy wires using standard flat electrodes. When welding light wires to heavy wires precautions should be taken against overheating and distorting the finer wire if the discrepancy in bulk is at all great. This means, in brief, using a grooved electrode to weld the fine wire and, if this is done, quite fine spring wires may be successfully attached to heavy archwires (*Fig.* 232). When making such a weld it is not in fact necessary to do more than make a fine V groove in the tip of the upper electrode with the edge of a fine jeweller's file to accommodate the fine wire. Sufficient adaptation of the electrode to the curve of the wire is achieved in this way. When grooving an electrode to fit heavier wires it is desirable to make the groove with a very fine fissure bur. For the most perfect results the electrode should be made to fit each size of wire as accurately as possible.

This would mean having a large selection of electrodes with a different size of groove in each. It is found that it is not in practice essential to have such a series of grooved

0·9-mm., 0·8-mm., 0·7-mm., and even 0·6-mm. thickness. Although the hollow of the electrode does not fit all these wires perfectly, the fact that the electrode is grooved at all protects

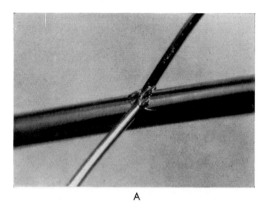

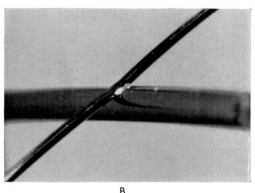

A   B

Fig. 232.—**A**, 0·3-mm. wire welded to 1·0-mm. arch, using flat electrodes. The fine spring wire has been overwelded and crushed. A degree of welding power that does not injure the outer surface of the fine wire is also insufficient to produce an adequate weld at all. **B**, The upper electrode has been grooved and now a secure weld can be made without distorting the fine wire.

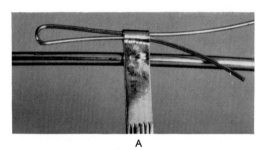

A

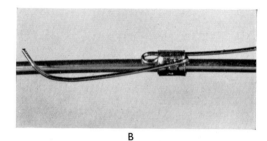

B

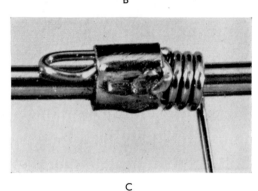

C

Fig. 233.—The welded tape loop for attaching fine spring wires. **A**, A loop of tape 2·5-mm. × 0·15-mm. is pulled up tightly on the fine (0·3-mm.) spring wire (*see Fig.* 91). The tape loop is welded to the heavy archwire. **B**, The tape loop is cut off and welded to the arch again close up to but not through the fine spring wire. The wire loop is then pulled up by the short end into the tape loop until jamming occurs and the short tail of wire turned tightly back. **C**, The short tail is cut off and smoothed, the tape welds and cut ends are smoothed, and the auxiliary spring is wound. Note how the pull of winding the spring is against the loop of the tape and not against the weld. This attachment is suitable for any fine apron spring. Even when coils are not wanted, one or two turns of the spring wire are taken around the arch.

electrodes to fit all the heavier wires. If an electrode is grooved to fit a 1·0-mm. wire accurately, it will be found that this groove will work very satisfactorily with wires of

the wires in the way that has been already discussed. For the finer wires, 0·5-mm. and smaller, a finer groove should be made in the electrode with a fine file as mentioned above.

156

Another method for overcoming the problem of attaching a very fine wire to a heavy arch is to make an attachment with a small strap or loop of tape, so avoiding actually welding the fine wire. The tape can be easily welded to the arch wire making a strong joint (*Fig.* 233).

The practice of reinforcing welded joints with solder is to be deprecated. A properly welded joint does not need any reinforcement. Once the parts have been welded, it is virtually impossible to solder them properly as small extrusions of metal which are tarnished prevent the flow of solder into the interstices of the joint. It is far better to develop the potentialities of both methods to the full and either to weld or to solder. Each method has its own sphere of usefulness and for certain purposes either method may be used, but the use of both together is never necessary and rarely produces the best result.

CHAPTER XIV

THE SOLDERING OF STAINLESS STEEL FOR REMOVABLE APPLIANCE CONSTRUCTION

THE use of soldered joints* in stainless steel for orthodontic appliances brings with it certain technical difficulties. Firstly, no union takes place between solder and steel and as a result the solder, under the conditions of stress and strain found in the mouth and the action of the oral secretions, is liable to come away from the steel, leading to joint failure. Secondly, the heating of stainless steel to the temperature required for soldering anneals the steel and makes it useless for spring purposes at the annealed part. Heat treatment does not restore elasticity to the metal.

In the construction of removable appliances, soldering almost always refers to the soldering of wires, and here the two difficulties referred to can be overcome by good design of the joint and by accurate control of heat distribution during the soldering operation.

JOINT DESIGN

Wherever possible wires should be joined by turning one wire around the other and soldering the joint. This may seem a clumsy method, but the joint so formed is much more reliable than one formed by simply crossing the wires and soldering. The extra bulk formed by turning one wire around the other can be allowed for, and in some instances can be used to advantage as, for instance, in the stop hook for intermaxillary and extra-oral traction. It will be noted, too, that in the construction of the extra-oral attachment for cervical traction to a removable upper appliance, a 1·25-mm. wire was bound to a 1·00-mm. wire with 0·3-mm. soft stainless steel wire and the whole joint then soldered. This method is useful in certain cases.

Where a simple crossed or lapped joint is unavoidable, this may be made, of course, and good results are obtainable if the other principles of joint construction are attended to.

It is important, when soldering wires, to encase the joint completely in solder. The solder on the outer aspects of the joint will be thin; but however thin, the solder must be present all round the joint. The mechanical continuity of the solder has much to do with the permanence of the joint. For this reason soldered joints should not be polished; polishing removes the outer layer of solder and exposes the wire. This makes a break in the continuity of the solder which, in the mouth, generally leads to failure of the joint. Flux should be removed from soldered joints when the joint has barely cooled, by picking it away with a probe; the solder will be found to have a bright, smooth surface which is perfectly clean and hygienic. It is not usually feasible or necessary to remove flux on soldered joints on appliances by boiling it off with alum solution.

HEAT CONTROL

The most convenient method of melting solder for stainless steel soldering is by means of the miniature blowlamp which burns coal-gas and compressed air. The air jet in the blowlamp should be small enough to make it possible to produce a fine needle flame 1 cm. long when required. If the air jet is found to be too coarse, it may be bushed with stainless steel tubing, using 0·5-mm. internal tubing as the final jet size. Only low-pressure compressed air is required, but the importance of having a steady air pressure cannot be stressed too much. The imposition on the operator of the responsibility of blowing the

---

* Suitable materials for soldering stainless steel wire are "Easy-flo" silver brazing alloy 0·025 in. wireform and "Easy-flo" flux powder. Johnson, Matthey & Co. Ltd.

flame increases the difficulty of an already delicate operation. It is much better to make the soldering flame one of the constant factors in the operation by using compressed air to produce a jet.

Only enough heat should be used to melt the solder and the use of a fierce flame should be avoided. A soft, quiet blue flame will melt solder quite adequately and give the operator time to observe the flow of the solder and manipulate the wires. Even slight overheating of a joint produces burning of the wire and the solder, a weak joint, and a rough pitted surface on the solder. The control of heat application in soldering stainless steel is critical, as is also the manipulation of the wires and the application of the solder.

The final soldering operation should be performed if possible in one heating. Re-melting a joint to add more solder or make adjustments increases the risk of burning the solder and the wire.

The localization of heat to the site of soldering is important when it is wished to avoid annealing a large section of wire, and where wires embedded in baseplates are being soldered. Heat may be localized by covering the adjoining wires with wet napkins or cotton-wool, or other blanketing material; by using a small flame; or by soldering rapidly and quenching the joint in cold water so that heat does not get time to travel down the wires. Another method of heat control is to melt solder on a separate piece of wire and to touch the wires to be soldered against the molten bead of solder. The molten solder will then flow on to the joint. This method provides both heat control and control of the amount of solder to be applied to a joint.

The annealing of stainless steel wire during soldering operations is related to two distinct uses of the wire. Firstly wires which are used as rigid arches, for example free sliding buccal arches, do not suffer from annealing because the wire is still strong enough when softened to resist the pressures of the forces applied to it. The same applies to wires, usually 0·7-mm. soft, used for hooks. Such wires are strong enough even when soft to withstand the pressure of intermaxillary traction. Secondly,

finer wires used for springs, when annealed, become quite useless for their purpose. It is necessary when attaching such wires by soldering to use only enough heat to melt the solder, so annealing as little of the spring wire as possible, and to wind the annealed part of

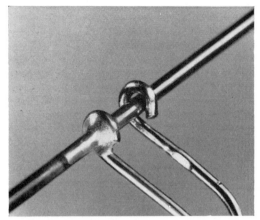

Fig. 234.—Soldering medium wire to thick. The medium wire is turned around the thick wire (right) and the loop soldered.

any such spring around the arch before beginning to use the wire as a spring. If it is possible to use the turns of such a spring wire around the arch as the coils of the spring, so much the better. The annealed part of the wire will then be well out of the way and unlikely to break down.

OTHER POINTS IN SOLDERING

If solder is first of all flowed around one or both of the wires to be soldered and the wires held in position, a gentle heat just enough to melt the solder will produce a perfect joint.

Flux must be applied liberally at all stages of stainless steel soldering. The flux/water mixture has a tendency to boil and leave areas of metal uncovered. This may be avoided by drying on a thick layer of flux by gentle heat before heating to soldering temperature and by cleaning just the area to be soldered with a fine cuttlefish disk or a fine smooth file. A wire so prepared will take a smooth and even layer of flux which remains evenly spread when molten. For small joints between wires it is not necessary to prepare the wire apart from wiping off surface dirt or grease. Stainless steel soldering takes place in a bath of molten flux which protects the metal and the solder from oxidization.

Soldering Medium Wires to Thick Wires.— The medium thick wire is turned accurately

the joint is uniformly covered with solder (*Fig.* 235 B). The wires are withdrawn from the flame and held until the solder hardens.

If required, such wires as these or wires of equal thickness may be united without looping one about the other. It is necessary to make

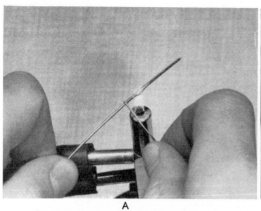
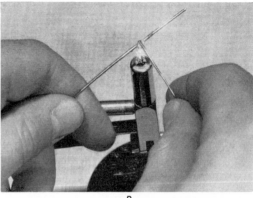

A   B

Fig. 235.—Soldering medium wire to thick. **A**, A blob of solder is melted on the thick wire; **B**, The looped wire slid into the molten solder and held for a second until the joint is complete. The joint may be soldered in one heating if necessary.

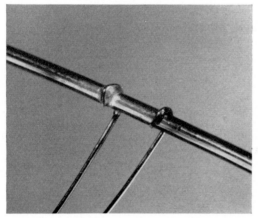

Fig. 236.—Soldering thin wire to thick. Right, fine wire clipped on to thick; left, the joint soldered.

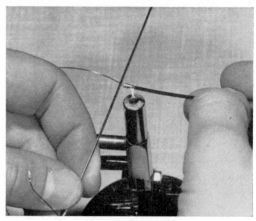

Fig. 237.—Soldering thin wire to thick. A piece of 1·25-mm. wire with solder on the end is heated in a fine flame and the molten solder touched on to the fine and thick wires which are clipped together; the solder will then flow on to the joint without overheating the fine wire.

around the thick wire, but not so tightly that it will not slide along the thick wire (*Fig.* 234). A bead of solder is melted on to the thick wire at the site of the joint (*Fig.* 235 A). The thinner wire is fluxed and brought near to the solder bead, which is again melted, and the loop in the thin wire is moved into the molten solder and heating continued for a second or so until

sure that the wires are completely encased in solder. Do not polish the joint.★

★ This method of soldering was described by Mr. Harold G. Watkin in the *Transactions of the British Society for the Study of Orthodontics* in the discussion of the paper by Mr. R. Cutler (1932).

Soldering Fine Wires to Thick Wires.—The fine wire is given slightly more than a half turn at the extreme end and clipped on to the thick wire at the site of the joint and both wires fluxed all round (*Fig.* 236). A piece of 1·25-mm. wire is filed flat across the end and

chipped off and the fine wire wound at least once completely around the thick arch, after which it may be used as a spring with or without further coils. By this technique it is possible to solder a 0·3-mm. wire to a 1·0-mm. wire without softening the 0·3-mm. wire.

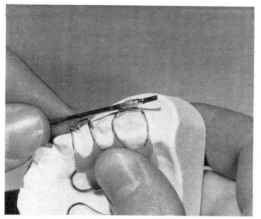

Fig. 238.—Soldering tubes to clasps. The tube is coated with solder and alinement tested.

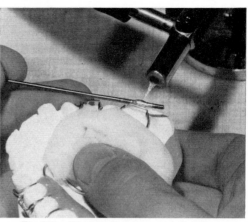

Fig. 239.—The baseplate is protected with a wet napkin and heat applied to the solder on the tube only, with a fine needle-pointed flame.

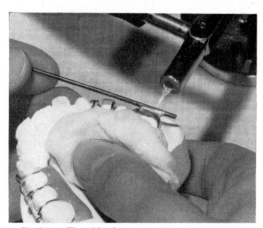

Fig. 240.—The solder flows around the clasp wire without the necessity of heating the wire itself.

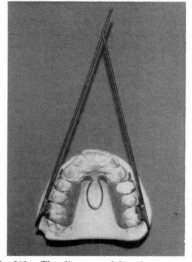

Fig. 241.—The alinement of the tubes is simplified by using long lengths and allowing these to cross anteriorly.

a small spot of solder is melted on to the tip. This piece of wire is heated with a small, fine, fairly fierce flame just proximal to the bead of solder, which melts. The wires to be joined are held against the molten solder, which transfers itself to them without overheating the fine wire (*Fig.* 237). The wires are withdrawn from the flame and when cool the flux is

The soldering of tubes to Adams clasps is strictly comparable to the joining of wires by soldering, and all the same considerations have to be taken into account.

161

A long length of tubing should be used, and the required section cut off after soldering. If it is desired to use up short lengths of tubing, these may be alined and held in position by

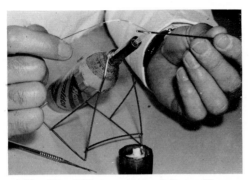

Fig. 242.—Soldering with bottled gas. The gas container and burner are supported at a suitable angle in a wire or wooden cradle. The gas container and burner are the Flamidor Butagaz system of French origin but available on most continents.

placing them on a longer length of finer tubing, or straight wire.

The area of tube to be soldered is coated with a thick blob of solder (*Fig.* 238), and the tube tried on the appliance for alinement. The model on which the appliance was processed is preserved and used to assist in the alinement of the tubes.

The bridge of the clasp is then fluxed and, using a very fine needle-pointed flame, the solder on the tube is heated, when it will flow on to and around the wire of the clasp (*Figs.* 239, 240). It is most important that heat should be applied only to the solder on the tube by means of a fine short needle-pointed flame. If the wire of the clasp is heated, the tags will lose their hardness and the clasp will not then remain tight when adjusted. The baseplate is protected by a well-wetted napkin arranged to cover it completely opposite the clasp and the two adjoining teeth.

The tubing must be alined to suit the curve of the arch in the buccal segments, and also in the horizontal plane to suit the level at which the bow being used must lie anteriorly. When one tube has been soldered, the alinement of the second in the horizontal plane is greatly facilitated, as the two lengths of tubing will cross anteriorly (*Fig.* 241), and it is only

162

necessary to consider the alinement of this tube in a bucco-lingual direction.

The soldering of tubes to premolar clasps is done in exactly the same way. A little less solder is required and it is not spread as far along the tube.

The author finds it most convenient when soldering tubes to have the flame coming towards him, as, holding the model and tubing in this way, it is easier to judge the alinement of the tube. There is a risk of burning the fingers or clothing accidentally, however, and others may prefer to have the flame pointing in the opposite direction.

For the sake of clarity in the illustrations flux has been omitted in all the soldering operations. Flux must, of course, be applied liberally as mentioned earlier.

The practice of welding the parts together before soldering does not always confer the advantage of a doubly strong joint and may in fact lead to trouble in the long run. Welding parts together inevitably leads to some oxidizing of the metal and the formation of small gaps and crevices between the parts which are difficult to clean out and flux properly and into which solder will not readily flow. Both these factors are inimical to the creation of a properly soldered joint, and if the first attempt at soldering is not successful subsequent re-heating may only make matters worse.

Soldering with Butane Gas.—The most easily regulated flame for various soldering operations is that obtained with coal gas and compressed air using a miniature blowlamp. In areas where a town gas supply or compressed air are not available, fine soldering may be done using a small jeweller's blowlamp designed to run on miniature butane gas bottles (*Fig.* 242).

The burner is simply screwed on to the gas bottle and this releases the gas which burns as a fine blue jet. When the burner is unscrewed the gas bottle is re-sealed.

When using the butane burner it will be found that the flame is fairly hot and cannot be turned up or down. With a little practice it will be found possible to regulate the heating effect on different sizes of materials by positioning the parts to be soldered in different areas of the flame.

CHAPTER XV

AN ORTHODONTIC COIL SPRING WINDER

Coil springs find a great variety of uses both in fixed and removable orthodontic appliance technique, and it is important, therefore, to have at hand a rapid and reliable method of forming these springs in different diameters and different gauges of wire. The winder that is

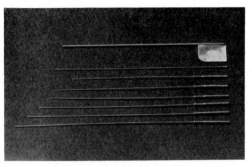

Fig. 243.—Winding jig, lining tube, and six winding mandrels sizes 1·0 mm., 0·9 mm., 0·8 mm., 0·7 mm., 0·6 mm., and 0·5 mm. thick. The mandrels are graduated in length from thickest to thinnest, so that selection of the required size is facilitated.

illustrated in this paper has been in use for many years at the Eastman Dental Hospital, London, where it was introduced by Mr. J. S. Beresford. The inspiration for this device came originally from a winder, identical in principle but rather different in design, described by Lowrie J. Porter (1941, 1943). The present author has made a few small modifications to the East-man pattern that make for greater ease in con-struction and speed in operation, but does not claim any originality for the device as a whole.

The winder consists essentially of a series of mandrels made of stainless steel wire from 0·5 mm. to 1·0 mm. thick, on which the coils are wound. This range of diameters will cover all normal orthodontic coil spring require-ments. These mandrels run in a stainless steel tube, 1·0 mm. internal diameter, and the spring wire is fed in at right angles through a fine 0·5-mm. internal tube (Fig. 243). The spring

wire is attached to the mandrel temporarily by means of a perforated disk fixed to the mandrel through a hole in which the spring wire is passed (Fig. 244).

Construction of the Mandrels.—The mandrels are constructed from hard stainless steel wire,

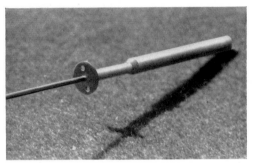

Fig. 244.—A mandrel showing the shank, made from a bur or straight handpiece mandrel with a disk 5–6 mm. diameter perforated in two places. One of these holes is used to retain the spring wire during winding of the spring.

straightened as well as possible and soldered on to a straight bur shank through the medium of a short length of tubing. The bur is first ground down at the end to a diameter of 1·0 mm. forming a short stub 3·0 mm. long with a definite shoulder at the junction with the bur shank (Fig. 245 A and B). This stub is most easily formed by holding the bur in a straight handpiece and, while running the bur rapidly, holding it against a fine, new carborundum wheel which is running on a lathe. If this wheel is reasonably new a definite sharp step can be formed where the stub projects from the bur shank.

A length of 1·0-mm. tubing is next fitted over the stub and soldered on. This tube is then cut off, leaving about 1·0 cm. attached to the bur shank. The piece of wire from which the mandrel is to be made is straightened and pushed into the open end of the tubing.

163

A piece of steel molar band material 5–6 mm. square and at least 0·15 mm. thick is perforated centrally with a hole of the same size as the mandrel wire and is slipped on to the wire and pushed right up against the tubing. Tube, wire, and band material are then soldered together using a minimum of solder and heat (*Fig.* 245 C).

An alternative method of constructing mandrels is to start with the conventional straight handpiece mandrel as used for sandpaper disks, discarding the central screw at the head (*Fig.* 246 A). The flange at the end is ground off (*Fig.* 246 B), and the winding wire fitted into the central hole with the square of

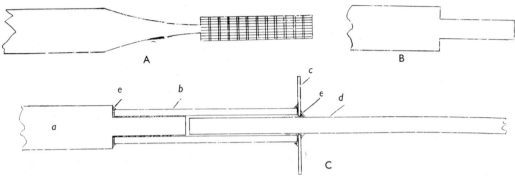

Fig. 245.—Construction of winding mandrel from straight handpiece bur shank. A, Bur, any kind can be used. B, Bur ground down forming stub 3–5 mm. long and 1·0 mm. thick. C, 1·0-mm. tubing soldered over stub. A long piece is used to facilitate soldering and tubing is then cut off leaving 1·0 cm. attached to bur (*a*, *b*). The winding wire (*d*) is then fitted in and a plate of stainless steel tape (*c*) is fitted over the wire and the whole soldered together (*e*).

It will be found that the finer mandrel wires are a rather slack fit in the tubing and may be a little eccentric when soldered in, but this does not affect the efficiency of the winder. When making the 0·5-mm. mandrel it is helpful to put a piece of 0·5-mm. tubing inside the 1·0-mm. tubing. This will centre the mandrel accurately.

The square plate of stainless steel is next turned into a circle by rotating the mandrel in a handpiece and holding the edge of the plate lightly against a rotating carborundum wheel. Two small holes are finally drilled in the disk with a spear point drill and the whole assembly smoothed off and polished.

It is helpful to make the set of mandrels of different lengths, the thickest being the longest, each successively thinner mandrel being shorter by 1·0 cm. or ½ in. A useful selection of mandrels is 1·0 mm. reducing by 0·1 mm. to 0·5 mm. thick, which is about the thinnest that it is practicable to use. This will give a set of six mandrels which may be selected at will by their lengths. The longest mandrel does not need to be longer than 10 in. overall, making it possible to wind a spring of about 8 in. in length if necessary.

tape in position and the mandrel, wire, and tape soldered together as before (*Fig.* 246 C). The complete mandrel is then finished off by rounding the square of tape into a circle, perforating, and smoothing off.

The Winding Jig.—The winding jig consists of a piece of 1·0-mm. internal stainless steel tube, 7–8 in. long, soldered to the long edge of a piece of 24 gauge stainless steel plate approximately 3 × 2 cm. in size. Along the adjoining edge of the plate is soldered a finer shorter length of tubing 0·5-mm. internal diameter (*Figs.* 243, 247). It is a great help if these pieces of tubing can be lightly tacked to the plate by welding before they are soldered. The alinement of these tubes and the relation of their ends should be carefully noted (*Figs.* 247, 248).

Use of the Winder.—The spring wire is fed through the fine tube until about 1·5 cm. project past the large tube. The mandrel is inserted past the fine wire into the large tube and pushed in until the disk is approaching the projecting end of the spring wire. The spring wire is bent over and led through one of the holes in the disk and the mandrel pushed right home. About 1 cm. of spring wire should project through the hole in the disk. The mandrel is then put into a straight handpiece and the engine set in motion, when the coils will become wound on the mandrel (*Fig.* 249). It is necessary to control the rate at which the mandrel is withdrawn from the tube

Some operators prefer to wind wire directly off the spool on to the coil winder. This method is not always suitable when spools of wire are kept in a dispenser, and it is found to be much more satisfactory to remove a length of wire, 1–2 ft. in length, and to use this for coil winding. The entry of the wire into the feeder

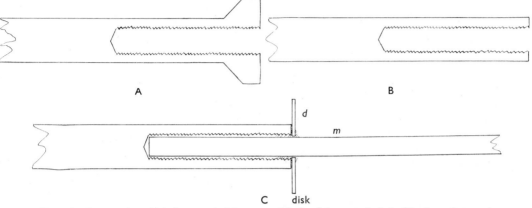

Fig. 246.—Construction of winding mandrel from a straight handpiece mandrel, A. The flange is ground off, B. The plate of stainless steel *d* and winding wire *m* are fitted as in *Fig.* 245 and soldered together.

to prevent either an open coil being wound or the coil wire from riding over coils already formed and jamming the winder.*

The most generally useful way of winding coil springs is to wind them all closely, that is with all the coils touching each other. Such coils are then "set" to give their optimum working range in compression by stretching the spring by its extreme ends an adequate amount. The spring will be found to stretch perfectly uniformly. The spring is then replaced on the mandrel and compressed completely. When released the spring will be found to return to a certain point. The useful working range of the spring in compression lies between this point and total compression, because it is known that total compression will not deform the spring and that it will always return to the point from which it was compressed.

---

* It is most important when making coil springs to use only a dental surgery engine and *never* a laboratory engine. The surgery engine has accurate slow speeds needed for spring winding and can be stopped instantly if the wire becomes tangled or looped around a finger. Most laboratory engines are too fast and do not stop quickly when required.

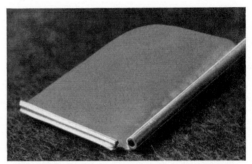

Fig. 247.—The relationship of the working ends of the winding tube (1·0 mm. internal diameter) and the feeder tube (0·5 mm. internal diameter).

tube can be controlled by passing the wire through the fingers of the left hand (*Fig.* 250). If the loops of unwound wire are allowed to hang loosely and a careful winding speed is used, there is no tendency for tangle to occur and the wire uncoils itself naturally as it passes through the fingers.

When winding springs on the 0·5-mm. mandrel, the mandrel is often found to be unstable inside the 1·0-mm. winding tube and difficulty may be experienced in obtaining a

165

smooth coil spring. The difficulty may be overcome by lining the 1·0-mm. tube with a length of 0·5-mm. internal tubing. The lining tube must be prevented from rotating and moving longitudinally inside the larger tube. This liner is stabilized by means of a cuff or clip of band material, welded or soldered

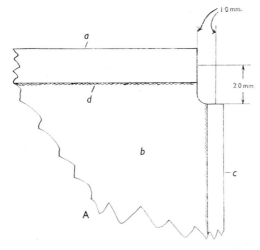

Removing the Spring from the Winder.— During the course of winding, the spring is bound tightly around the mandrel, which cannot be withdrawn from the spring while there is any wire still in the feed tube. The mandrel, spring, and jig can be separated in two ways:—

1. If the supply of spring wire runs out and the last of the wire is wound on to the mandrel,

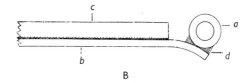

Fig. 248.—A, Plan of the arrangement of the ends of the winder and feeder tubes. The dimensions shown should be carefully observed to secure the best results. B, View of the winding tube, end on. Note that the edge of the plate is bent down so that the centre line of the feeder tube is level with the centre of the winding tube. It is then possible to wind springs in either direction with equal tension. *a*, Main or winding tube; *b*, Steel baseplate material; *c*, Feeder tube; *d*, Solder.

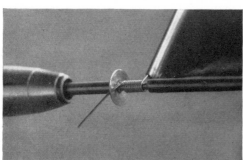

Fig. 249.—The winder in use. This spring is being wound in a right-handed manner. The mandrel may, however, be equally well rotated in the opposite direction.

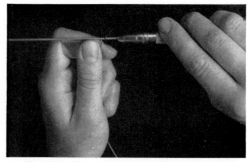

Fig. 250.—The winder in use. The spring wire is controlled by the fingers of the left hand. The wire can be seen entering from below. A slow winding speed should be used until experience has been gained in controlling the entry of the wire and withdrawal of the mandrel from the jig.

to the outer or far end of the liner, which clips over the outside of the outer end of the main winding tube. The construction of this part is shown in *Fig.* 251. When winding coils on the 0·5-mm. mandrel, therefore, the lining tube is slipped into the main winding tube and the clip or cuff steadies the fine tube in the larger one. At the inner or working end the lining tube must be quite flush with the outer tube and must not project.

the tension of the spring is released and the whole spring unwinds slightly and relaxes its grip on the mandrel. The mandrel can then be withdrawn from the jig and the spring pulled off the mandrel; the tail of wire projecting through the hole in the disk slips out perfectly easily.

2. If it is desired to withdraw the spring from the winder before the supply of wire has

run out, or in order to leave a coil spring with a tail of wire attached, it is important first to release the tension in the spring which is gripping the mandrel. This is done by releasing the grip of the handpiece on the shank of the mandrel. The spring and mandrel then unwind slightly and the grip of the spring

The thicker wires, 0·3 mm., 0·35 mm., and 0·4 mm., are more suitable for Trevor Johnson friction fit stops which are wound on a mandrel one size, or 0·1 mm., smaller than the arch on which they are to be used. The author finds that for these stops it is better to use a large number of coils of a fairly fine wire than a

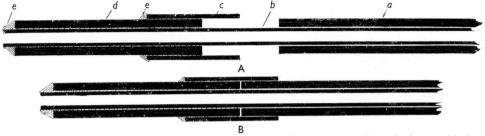

Fig. 251.—A, Section showing construction of the lining tube for the main winding tube for use with the 0·5-mm. mandrel. *a*, The main winding tube; *b*, The 0·5-mm. lining tube; *c*, A cuff of steel band material, soldered to the short length of 1·0-mm. tube; *d*, A short length of 1·0-mm. tube soldered to the lining tube at the end; *e*, Solder. B, The lining tube pushed home. The cuff of steel fits tightly over the winding tube, so steadying the lining tube. The other end of the lining tube is flush with the end of the outer tube.

on the mandrel is released. The mandrel is then pulled out and the spring is removed from the jig by drawing the unused portion of the spring wire, attached to the coil spring, through the feeder tube.

POINTS TO REMEMBER

Coil springs can be wound with this simple apparatus in wire from 0·45 mm. thick downwards on mandrels from 1·0 mm. thick downwards. It will naturally be found that it is not feasible to wind a thick wire on a thin mandrel; a point will be reached where the mandrel will not stand the strain or the engine used for driving the device will become overloaded. Up to this point, however, there is a very large range of coil springs that can be made using different combinations of thicknesses of wire and thicknesses of mandrel.

In practice, coil springs are generally made of wires 0·15 mm. or 0·2 mm. thick. Thicker wires give springs which are too powerful and have too short a range of action. For twin-wire arch coil springs, 0·15-mm. wire wound on a mandrel 0·5 mm. thick gives a very suitable spring. For springs of larger diameter, that is 0·8 mm., 0·9 mm., or 1·0 mm., wire of 0·2 mm. thickness may in certain circumstances be used.

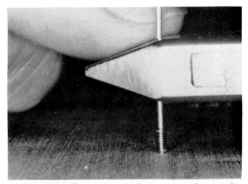

Fig. 252.—Pressing an archwire into a friction-fit stop. The archwire is tapered slightly at the end and is held in Adams pliers near to the end using the right hand. The end of the archwire is placed in the stop which is rested on a piece of soft wood. Using the left thumb on the pliers beaks the archwire is pressed into and through the stop.

small number of coils of a thicker wire, i.e., six turns of 0·3-mm. wire rather than two or three turns of 0·4-mm. wire. The former stop will be as firm as, but more resilient in itself and less likely to loosen in use than the latter. On the other hand, if the friction fit attachment is to be used also as traction hook by forming a free end into a hook, a firm wire must be used for the purpose of the hook and therefore a 0·4-mm. wire requires to be used for the whole attachment.

The winder can also be used for both right-hand and left-hand coils, a point that must be taken into consideration when the end of the wire is to be used for spring or hook purposes. A winder of this type once made up will last for years, the only replacement being possibly the occasional reconstruction of one of the finer mandrels should breakage occur.

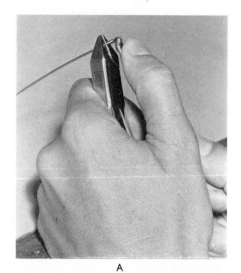

A

To place a stop on the archwire, the end of the arch is slightly tapered and pressed into the stop. To get the archwire through the stop the arch is gripped close to the stop with Adams universal pliers. The stop is placed on a block of wood and the pliers pressed firmly at the end near the archwire with the left thumb. The grip of the pliers on the archwire must not be allowed to slip and the end of the archwire will pass through the stop and into the wood (*Fig.* 252).

To move the stop along the archwire, the archwire is gripped in Adams pliers in the *left* hand, as shown in *Fig.* 253 A. The stop to be moved should only be a few millimetres from the pliers. The end of the archwire projecting through the stop is lightly held with

Fig. 253.—Positioning the stop on the archwire. A, The archwire is gripped in Adams pliers using the left hand. B, The stop is a short way from the pliers. This distance can be predetermined making accurate movements of a stop very easy. Note tapered end of 1·0-mm. archwire. C, Howe pliers are placed over the projecting end of the archwire which is held *lightly* using the right hand. Almost any other fine nosed pliers may be used as well as Howe's. The *left* thumb is placed on top of the Howe pliers and presses the stop along the archwire until it comes in contact with the Adams pliers.

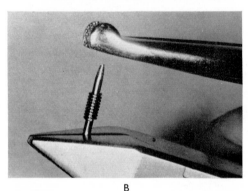

B

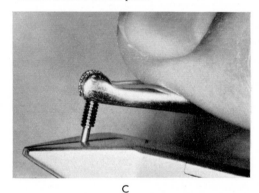

C

The Fitting and Adjustment of Friction Fit Stops.—Friction fit stops on heavy archwires, 1·0 mm. or 0·9 mm. in thickness, are a great convenience as they may be moved to any position on the archwire as required. The stops should consist of about six turns of 0·35 mm. hard wire wound on a mandrel 0·1 mm. smaller than the archwire being used.

pliers such as Howe pliers (*Fig.* 253 B, C) held in the *right* hand.

Using the left thumb (*Fig.* 253 A), the stop is pressed along the archwire, holding firmly with the left hand and lightly with the right.

By this method the stop can be moved easily and the amount of movement pre-determined by the point at which the archwire is held with the Adams pliers.

CHAPTER XVI

THE PREPARATION OF THE ORTHODONTIC STUDY MODEL*

STUDY models have always been and will remain one of the most informative records of the arrangement of the teeth and of the occlusion available to the orthodontist; no other method of recording can embody the three-dimensional effect that is required. It is important, therefore, always to employ a model preparation routine that will ensure that accurate, well-made and finished study casts can be prepared without drudgery and the expenditure of an undue amount of time.

When preparing models of the teeth for study, record, and measurement purposes, it is usual to make them with a bulk of plaster in addition to the teeth, palate, and alveolar processes so that bases can be formed. The bases make a background against which the arrangement of the teeth is judged. The bases of the casts should be shaped so as to avoid any outline or angulation that will suggest abnormalities of alinement or position of the teeth that do not in fact exist. If the posterior surfaces of the models are cut in the same vertical plane this serves to register the occlusal relationship of the dental arches and makes the models easier to handle and store.

It was at one time recommended that the base of the upper model should be carved so that its top surface corresponded with the Frankfurt plane (Simon, 1926). This resulted in the production of a rather tall and bulky set of study models, and as X-ray cephalometry has made it possible to relate the arrangement of the teeth and the occlusion to the face and head as a whole, it is no longer necessary to prepare study models which

incorporate facial landmarks in the plaster bases.

There is one anatomical landmark which does appear in all study models and which is invariably used in making visual assessments of the arrangement of the teeth in the upper arch. This is the median palatine raphe and its associated palatal rugæ. The middle line of the palate has always been used in estimating the symmetry of the upper arch and the amount of drift of permanent teeth that has taken place following the early loss of deciduous teeth. If the bases of study casts are cut so as to be symmetrical about the median palatine raphe of the upper model, the eye is greatly aided in judging the symmetry or lack of symmetry of the dental arches when looking at record models.

The relationship between the occlusal plane and the model base must also be considered. It is not necessary to register the relationship of the occlusal plane, as this can be measured on cephalometric X-ray films. Rather than attempt to embody some guess as to the inclination of the occlusal plane in a set of study casts, the purely arbitrary decision should be taken to make the occlusal plane parallel to the top surface of the upper model. For this purpose the occlusal plane is defined by the incisal edges of the incisor teeth and the occlusal surfaces of the last pair of molars in the upper dental arch.

EQUIPMENT

1. One electric plaster-trimming machine with a medium-grit, carborundum wheel, grit No. 60, is suitable for a general-purpose machine. The platform of the machine must be perfectly flat and at right angles to the surface of the grinding wheel. The sides of the platform must be straight and parallel and also

---

* The method of study model preparation described owes much to the method suggested by G. Northcroft, shown in *The Science and Practice of Dental Surgery*, London: Oxford University Press, 1931.

at right angles to the wheel. If large numbers of study casts are to be prepared for exhibition or photographing, it is a great convenience to have a second machine with a very fine wheel, grit No. 120. With this machine the cut surfaces can be polished so that no hand finishing

The small pieces of equipment can be made in the laboratory. The rubber T-piece is made of firm rubber sheet $\frac{1}{8}$ in.–$\frac{1}{4}$ in. thick and to the size and shape shown in *Fig.* 258. The set squares and symmetroscope are made of perspex sheet $\frac{1}{8}$ in. thick to the sizes and

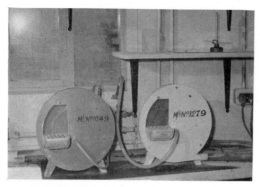

Fig. 254.—Two standard model-trimming machines. Medium grit on right; No. 120 grit on left. On the shelf above are surface gauge and symmetroscope.

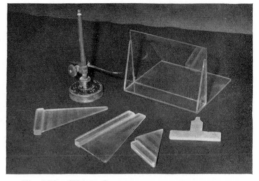

Fig. 255.—The surface gauge, symmetroscope, set squares, and the rubber T-piece.

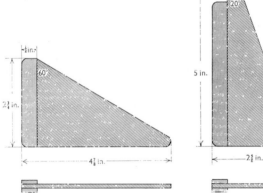

Fig. 256.—The set squares for trimming study models. These are made to the shapes and sizes shown, of $\frac{1}{8}$-in. perspex material cemented with chloroform.

or sandpapering is required on the cut surfaces. A very accurate, fine finish is produced in this way. One machine with a medium-grit wheel is all that is required for routine clinical purposes (*Fig.* 254).

2. One simple engineer's surface gauge.

3. One rubber T-piece, a symmetroscope, and three jigs for guiding the models to the correct angles, a piece of plate glass 10 in. square (*Figs.* 255–258).

shapes shown in *Figs.* 256, 257. On the viewing sheet of the symmetroscope the centre line and two sets of width lines are drawn with a fine needle and the lines filled in with indian ink (*Fig.* 257). The perspex can be sawn and filed to shape. If a heavy carpenter's plane and shooting board are used the truing up of the set squares is made easier. To put the set squares together, the pieces are clipped with clothes-pegs and chloroform run into the

170

joints by capillary attraction. The symmetroscope is similarly fixed together, and when the joints have dried they may be reinforced with a cement of perspex dissolved in chloroform.

STAGES IN THE PREPARATION OF STUDY MODELS

1. The Impression and Wax Bite.—The models should be cast in accurate impressions. To-day the alginate mixtures provide most

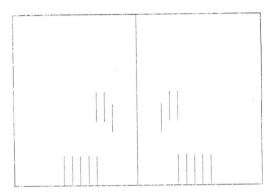

Fig. 257.—The screen of the symmetroscope measures 6 in. × 4 in. The markings are 5 mm. apart and are distributed symmetrically about the vertical centre line.

soft palate. Impressions which only take in the tooth crowns and a few millimetres of the adjoining gingival tissue are unsuitable for orthodontic record purposes. A wax bite should always be taken. This should consist of only a bar of moderately softened wax across the premolar region (*see Fig.* 262). When the teeth are fully closed, the molars will be in contact and the record models can easily be brought similarly into contact when registered in the wax bite. If a large area of

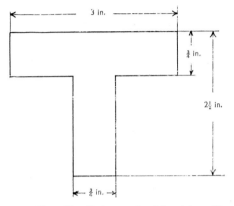

Fig. 258.—The rubber T-piece made of firm ⅛-in. rubber sheet.

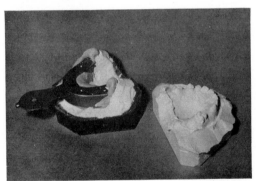

Fig. 259.—The models are cast in rubber formers. These provide a rough approximation to the shape of the base and give an adequate bulk of material for trimming.

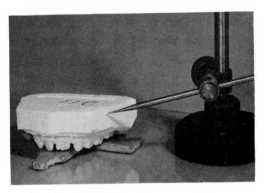

Fig. 260.—Scribing the upper model.

of the requirements of a good impression material. The impressions should extend to the limits of the buccal sulci and into the lingual sulcus in the molar region of the lower arch. The upper impression should cover the hard palate but should not extend on to the

wax covers the teeth it is difficult to bring the record models fully together. The wax should not be permitted to encroach on the incisors as the plaster reproductions of these teeth are easily broken off if the record casts are pressed into a wax bite. In some cases there are very few teeth in the buccal segments. In such cases, the wax bite bar must be thick enough to fill

171

the gaps in the buccal occlusion. When, later on, the record models are occluded and trimmed, there must be adequate support between the models in the premolar region so that no pressure is thrown on the incisors.

2. Casting the Model.—The models may be cast in plain dental plaster, in stone plaster, in plain-plaster–stone-plaster mixtures, or the teeth may be cast in stone plaster and the bases in plain plaster. The method of casting

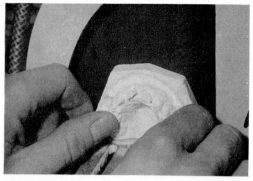

Fig. 261.—Trimming the base of the upper model to the correct depth.

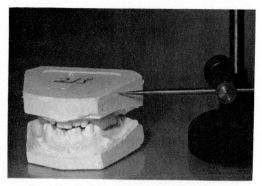

Fig. 262.—Scribing the base of the lower model. Note the size and position of the wax bite.

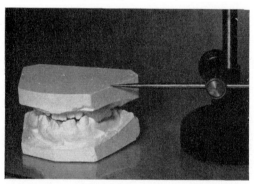

Fig. 263.—The lower model cut to correct depth. Note that the scribed line is still just visible.

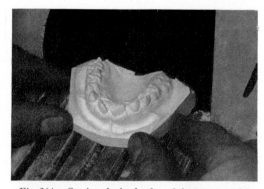

Fig. 264.—Cutting the back edge of the upper model.

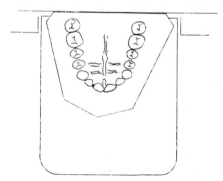

Fig. 265.—The back edge is trimmed at right angles to the middle line.

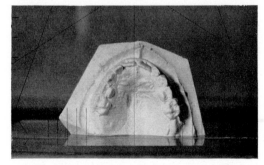

Fig. 266.—The upper model cut with the back edge at right angles to the middle line of the palate. Note that the centre line of the dental arch does not correspond with the middle line of the palate. |2 is missing.

is a matter of personal preference. Teeth cast in stone plaster are stronger than teeth cast in white plaster, but even stone plaster teeth will break if the study model is roughly handled. If plain plaster models are stored and treated with care they are completely satisfactory.

The models should be cast with sufficient plaster in the base to allow for trimming to shape. The use of rubber boxes greatly

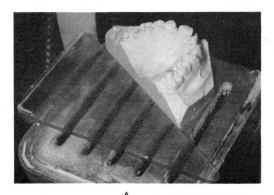
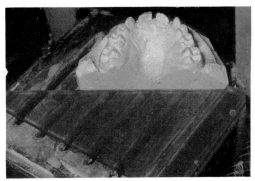

A   B

Fig. 267.—Trimming the front of the upper model. A, Right side; B, Left side.

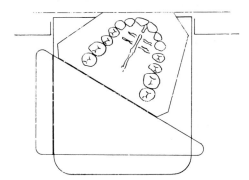
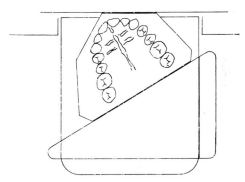

Fig. 268.—The front surfaces are cut so that the point of the model is in line with the middle line of the palate.

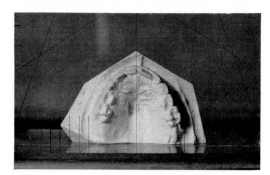

Fig. 269.—The point at the front of the model is in line with the centre line of the palate.

facilitates the casting of adequate bases with economy of plaster (*Fig.* 259).

3. Trimming the Bases.—

a. The upper model is set on the rubber T-piece on the plate glass and with the surface gauge a horizontal line is scribed right around the base of the model (*Fig.* 260).

b. The base of the model is trimmed to the scribed line (*Fig.* 261).

c. The models are placed in occlusion with the wax bite in position and placed on the glass plate, lower model uppermost. The base of the lower model is scribed all around parallel

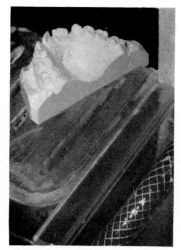

Fig. 270.—Trimming the left side of the model; the right side is similarly trimmed.

to the base of the upper and the lower is trimmed to the scribed line (*Figs.* 262, 263). The heights of the models must be determined by trial and standardized. A total height for deciduous teeth of 4 cm. and of 5 cm. for permanent teeth is suitable.

d. The heel or back surface of the upper model is trimmed back sufficiently and made at right angles to the median palatine raphe (*Figs.* 264–266).

e. The front of the model is trimmed so that the point is in line with the median palatine raphe (*Figs.* 267–269).

f. The sides of the model are trimmed equidistantly from the middle line, making the model of a suitable width (*Figs.* 270, 271).

g. The models are placed in occlusion with the wax bite in position and, using the upper

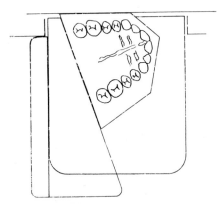
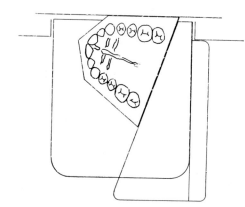

Fig. 271.—The sides of the model are cut symmetrically about the middle line.

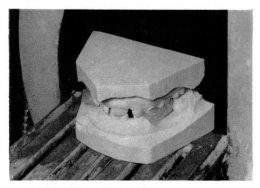

Fig. 272.—The upper model is used as a guide in trimming the back edge of the lower model.

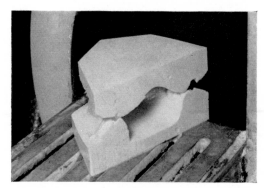

Fig. 273.—The upper model is used as a guide in trimming the sides of the lower model.

174

model as a guide, the heel or back surface and the sides of the lower model are trimmed to match the upper (*Figs.* 272, 273).

It is useful to use the second set square when trimming the sides of both models together.

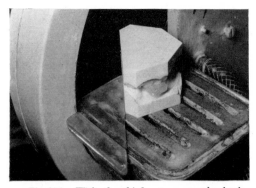

Fig. 274.—With the third set square the back corners of the upper and lower models are trimmed simultaneously.

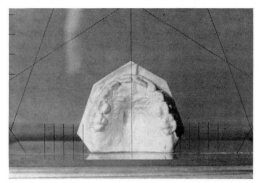

Fig. 276.—The upper model base is completely symmetrical.

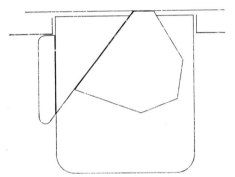
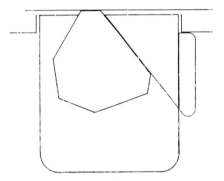

Fig. 275.—The distal corners are cut symmetrically to the middle line. This stage may conveniently be done with both models in occlusion so that upper and lower are cut simultaneously.

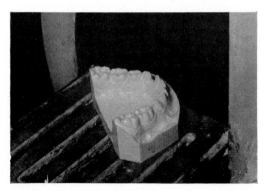

Fig. 277.—The front of the lower model is trimmed to a smooth curve

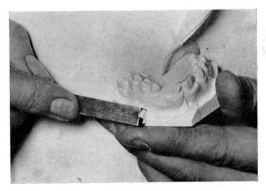

Fig. 278.—The rough edges are trimmed with a sharp vulcanite cutter.

175

h. The distal corners of the models are then trimmed, using the third set square (*Figs.* 274, 275) and the final symmetry of the upper model is checked (*Fig.* 276).

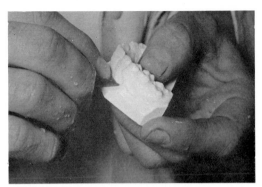

Fig. 279.—The curved cut edges are smoothed with wet and dry sandpaper.

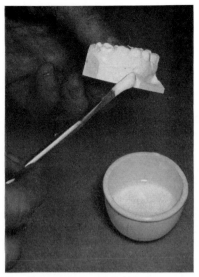

Fig. 280.—Air bubbles are filled with the smooth plaster mixture.

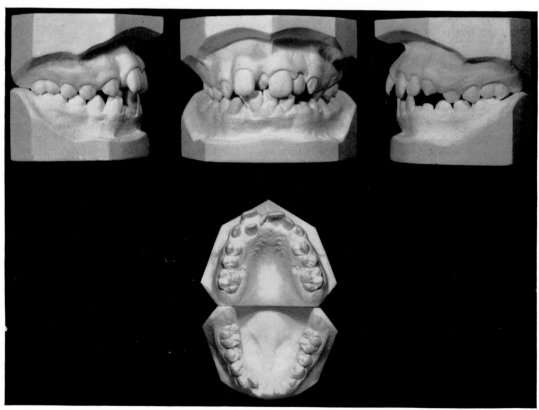

Fig. 281.—Photographs showing the models to best advantage.

176

i. The front of the lower model is trimmed to a curve to approximate the curve of the lower labial segment (*Fig.* 277).

j. The cut edges of the plaster are trimmed to smooth curves with a sharp hand chisel (*Fig.* 278).

k. For an exhibition or photographic finish the ground surfaces are polished on a No. 120 grit carborundum wheel. (If models are to be so treated only occasionally, the same effect can be produced by rubbing the models, in occlusion, on a very fine carborundum whetstone under a running tap.) The chiselled curves are smoothed with a scrap of well-wetted wet and dry sandpaper (*Fig.* 279). Any defects in the cut and polished surfaces due to air bubbles are filled with a creamy paste of plaster wiped on with a spatula and smoothed with the moist finger tip (*Fig.* 280).

Models are shown to the best advantage in photographs by reproducing left, central, and right views in occlusion and the occlusal view of both models (*Fig.* 281).

CARE OF RECORD MODELS

Record models should be dried out in a warm atmosphere or in a drying cabinet. The patient's name and number and the date on which the impressions were taken are most easily put on with a soft lead pencil. These details are best put on the top of the upper model and bottom of the lower. If put on the front and sides, such data may be difficult to eliminate from photographic reproductions. Record casts should be kept in boxes holding 5–6 sets of models, each pair held together by a light elastic band. A square of thin plastic foam should be placed between the occlusal surfaces of the teeth (*Fig.* 282). The wax bite should *not* be left between the teeth. In time the wax may stick to the plaster and pull pieces off the occlusal surfaces of the teeth when the models are separated. As the back

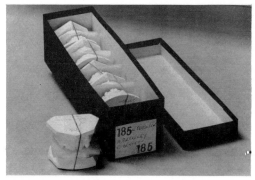

Fig. 282.—Models are best stored in long boxes 3 in.×3 in.×11 in. Sheet plastic foam is put between the occlusal surfaces.

surfaces or heels are cut exactly in the same vertical plane, the correct occlusion is best found by putting the models, back surfaces down, on a smooth flat surface and sliding them together. In most cases the wax bite has served its purpose and may be thrown away. In some cases where there are few teeth in the buccal segments and a thick wax bite has been taken, the wax should be stored with the models as it will be of help in finding the occlusal relationship at a later date.

BIBLIOGRAPHY

ADAMS, C. P. (1969), "An Investigation into Indications for and the Effects of the Function Regulator", *Trans. europ. orthod. Soc.*

ANDRESEN, V. (1936), "The Norwegian System of Functional Gnatho-orthopaedics", *Acta gnath., Kbh.*, **1**, No. 1.

BACKOFEN, W. A., and GALES, G. F. (1952), "The Low Temperature Heat Treatment of Stainless Steel", *Angle Orthodont.*, **21**, 117–124; also *Amer. J. Orthodont.*, **38**, 755–765.

BADCOCK, J. H. (1911), "The Screw Expansion Plate", *Trans. Brit. Soc. Orthodont.*, May–Dec., 3–8.

BEGG, P. R. (1965), *Begg Orthodontic Theory and Technique*. Philadelphia: W. B. Saunders.

BELL, R. DAVIDSON (1932), "Electric Resistance Spot Welding", *Dent. Rec.*, **52**, 554–566.

BJÖRK, A. (1963), Personal communication.

CHARLIER, M. (1928), "La Technique des Alliages inoxydables et celle de leur Sourdure électrique", *Odontologie*, **67**, 645–651.

COFFIN, WALTER H. (1881), "A Generalized Treatment of Irregularities", *Trans. Int. Congr. Med.*, 7th Session, London, Aug., vol. III, 542–547.

DE COSTER, L. (1931a), "Une Technique systématique d'Appareillage orthodontique en Acier inoxydable", *Province Dentaire*, **17**, 201–222, No. 4.

— — (1931b), "The Use of Rustless Steel in Dentofacial Orthopaedics", *Int. orthodont. Congr.*, **2**, 475–479; also in *Int. J. Orthodont.*, 1932, **18**, 1191–1195.

COUSINS, A. J. P. (1962), "Removable Appliance Technique: The Application of Rapid Cold-cure Acrylic Resin", *Dent. Practit.*, **13**, 29–32.

CROZAT, G. B. (1920), "Possibilities and Use of Removable Labiolingual Spring Appliances", *Int. J. Orthodontia*, **6**, 1.

CUTLER, R. (1932), "A New Preparation of British Stainless Steel", *Trans. Brit. Soc. Orthodont.*

DONDERS (1953), "Siehe bei Eckert-Möbius: normale und pathologische Physiologie der Nasen und Mundatmung", *Dtsch. Zahn-, Mund- u. Kieferheilk.*, **18**, 348.

DUYZINGS, J. A. C. (1954), *Orthodontische Apparatur*, pp. 33, 35, 37. Amsterdam: Dental-Depôt A. M. Disselkoen.

ECKERT-MÖBIUS (1962), "Grenzprobleme der Zahn-Mund- und Kieferheilkunde und der Hals-, Nasen- und Ohrenheilkunde aus rhinologischer Sicht", *Dtsch. Zahn-, Mund- u. Kieferheilk.*, **37**, 217.

— — (1963), "Grundsätzliches zur Atmung als rhinologisch-kieferorthopädisches Problem", *Acta oto-laryng., Stockh.*, Suppl. **183**, 36.

ENDICOTT, C. L., PEDLEY, V. G., and GROSSMANN, W. (1947), "Practical and Theoretical Observations on the Norwegian System", *Trans. Brit. Soc. Orthodont.*, 31–60.

FRÄNKEL, R. (1964), "Luftdruck, Atmung und die orofazialen Weichteile", *Dtsch. Zahn-, Mund- u. Kieferheilk.*, **43**, 367.

— — (1966), "The Theoretical Concept Underlying Treatment with Function Correctors", *Trans. europ. orthod. Soc.*, 233–250.

FRÄNKEL, R. (1966), *Funktionskieferorthopädie und der Mundvorhof als Apparative Basis*. Berlin: Verlag Volk und Gesundheit.

FRIEL, E. S. (1933), "The Practical Application of Stainless Steel in the Construction of Fixed Orthodontic Appliances", *Trans. Brit. Soc. Orthodont.*

— — and McKEAG, H. T. A. (1939), "The Design and Construction of Fixed Orthodontic Appliances in Stainless Steel", *Dent. Rec.*, **59**, 359–390; also *Trans. europ. orthod. Soc.*, 1938, **22**, 53–84.

FUNK, A. C. (1951), "The Heat Treatment of Stainless Steel", *Angle Orthodont.*, **21**, 129–138.

GRUDE, ROLF (1938), "The Norwegian System of Orthodontic Treatment", *Dent. Rec.*, **58**, 529–551.

HALLETT, G. E. M. (1952), "Cold Curing Acrylic Resin as an Aid in Orthodontics", *Brit. dent. J.*, **92**, 294–295.

HÄUPL, K., GROSSMANN, W. J., and CLARKSON, P. (1952), *Textbook of Functional Jaw Orthopaedics*. London: Kimpton.

HILL, C. V. (1954), "Controlled Tooth Movement. Multiband Round Arch Technique", *Dent. Practit.*, **5**, 2–13, 52–63.

HOPKIN, G. B. (1958), "The Rubber Peg Plate", *Trans. Brit. Soc. Orthodont.*, 86–87; also *Dent. Practit.*, **9**, 86–87.

JACKSON, V. H. (1904), *Orthodontia and Orthopedia of the Face*. Philadelphia: J. B. Lippincott.

— — (1906), "Orthodontia", *Dent. Cosmos*, **48**, 278.

JOHNSON, J. E. (1938), "The Twin-wire Appliance", *Amer. J. Orthodont.*, **24**, 303–327.

— — (1941), "The Construction and Manipulation of the Twin-wire Arch Mechanism", *Ibid.*, **27**, 289–307.

JOHNSON, W. TREVOR (1952), "A Friction Fit Attachment", *Trans. Brit. Soc. Orthodont.*, 65–69; also *Dent. Rec.*, **73**, 326–330.

KÖRBITZ, A. (1914), *Kursus der systematischen Orthodontik*, 2nd ed. Leipzig: Verlag H. Licht.

KORKHAUS, G. (1960), "Present Orthodontic Thought in Germany. Experiences with the Norwegian Method of Functional Orthopaedics in the Treatment of Distocclusion", *Amer. J. Orthodont.*, **46**, 270–287.

LAGER, H. (1963), Personal communication.

LEECH, H. LESTER (1951), "Appliances in the Treatment of the Collapsed Lower Arch", *Trans. Brit. Soc. Orthodont.*, 94–98.

McCALLIN, S. G. (1954), "Retraction of Maxillary Teeth with Removable Appliances using Inter-maxillary or Extra-oral Traction", *Dent. Rec.*, **74**, 36–41.

McCOY, J. D. (1941), *Applied Orthodontics*. London: Kimpton.

McKEAG, H. T. A. (1921), "Orthodontic Education", *Trans. Brit. Soc. Orthodont.*, 9–13.

— — (1928), "Physical Laws and the Design of Orthodontic Appliances", *Ibid.*, 69.

— — (1935), "The Teaching of Appliance Design in Orthodontia", *Ibid.*, 260–277.

MOSS, M. L. (1962), "Cephalometric Changes during Functional Appliance Therapy", *Trans. europ. orthod. Soc.*, 327–341.

179

NOLTEMEIER, H. (1949), *Einführung in die allgemeine Kiefer- und Gesichtsorthopädie*, vols. I, II. Alfeld: Buchdruckerei P. Dobler.

OLIVER, O. A.. IRISH, R. E., and WOOD, C. R. (1940), *Labiolingual Technique*. London: Kimpton.

PACKHAM, A. L. (1932) in Discussion on paper by CUTLER, R. (q.v.).

PARFITT, G. J., and FRIEL, E. S. (1946), "Experimental Welder Design", *Trans. Brit. Soc. Orthodont.*, 106; also *Dent. Rec.*, **67**, 250–259.

PORTER, LOWRIE J. (1941), "Johnson Twin Arch Technique", *Amer. J. Orthodont.*, **27**, 577–583.

— — (1943), *Ibid.*, **29**, 352.

ROBERTS, G. H. (1956), "A Removable Incisor Retractor", *Dent. Practit.*, VI, **7**, 220–1.

ROBIN, P. (1902), "Observations sur un nouvel Appareil de Redressement", *Rev. Stomat.*, *Paris*.

ROSSI, E. BONIFACE (1954), *Welding Engineering*. New York: McGraw-Hill.

ROUX, W. (1895), "Funktionelle Anpassung", *Real-Enzyklopädie der gesamten Heilkunde*, Bd. 8.

SCHWARZ, A. M. (1931), "Tissue Changes incidental to Orthodontic Tooth Movement", *Internat. orthodont. Congr.*, pp. 123–144.

SCHWARZ, A. M. (1954), *Die Zahn-, Mund- und Kieferheilkunde*, pp. 450–457. Munich: Urban.

— — (1956), *Lehrgand der Gebissnegelung*, II. Munich: Urban.

SIMON, P. (1926), "On the Necessity of Gnathostatic Diagnosis in Orthodontic Practice", *Int. J. Orthod.*, **12**, 1102–1113.

SOFTLEY, J. W. (1953), "Cephalometric Changes in Seven 'Post-normal' Cases treated by the Andresen Method", *Dent. Rec.*, **73**, 485–494.

STRANG, R. H. W. (1950), *A Textbook of Orthodontia*. London: Kimpton.

SVED, A. (1952), "Application of Engineering Methods to Orthodontics", *Amer. J. Orthodont.*, **38**, 399–421.

WATRY, F. M. (1947), "A Contribution to the History of Physiotherapeutics in Maxillofacial Orthopedics", *Trans. europ. orthod. Soc.*, 56.

WEBER, F. N. (1960), Personal communication.

WHITE, T. C., GARDINER, J. H., and LEIGHTON, B. C. (1954), *Orthodontics for Dental Students*. London: Staples.

WILD, N. (1950), "Design and Behaviour of Orthodontic Springs", *Trans. Brit. Soc. Orthodont.*, 109.

WILSON, H. E. (1953), "Myofunctional Appliances", *Dent. Practit.*, **4**, 70–78.

INDEX